The **Mind Body** Workout

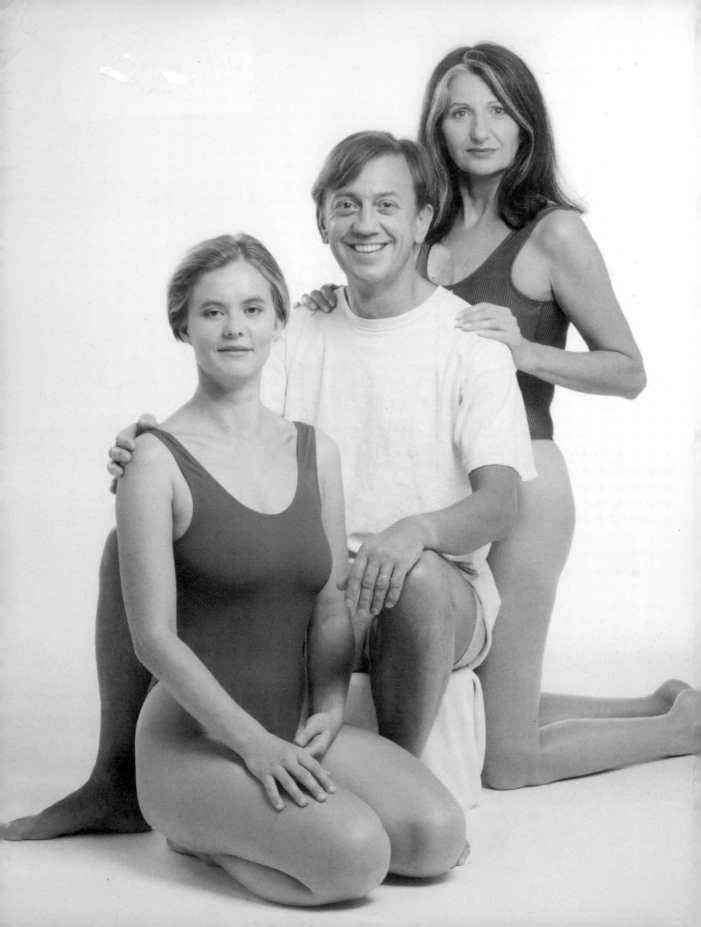

The **Mind Body** Workout

Lynne Robinson
and Helge Fisher

MACMILLAN

ADVICE TO THE READER

Before following any medical, dietary or exercise
advice contained in this book, it is recommended
that you consult your doctor if you suffer from
any health problems or special conditions or are
in any doubt as to its suitability.

First published 1998 by Pan Books
an imprint of Macmillan Publishers Ltd
25 Eccleston Place, London SW1W 9NF
and Basingstoke

Associated companies throughout the world

ISBN 0 330 36946 6

9 8 7 6 5 4 3 2 1

A CIP catalogue record for this book is available
from the British Library.

Typeset by SX Composing DTP, Rayleigh, Essex
Printed and bound in Great Britain by
Butler & Tanner, Frome and London

Contents

Explorations & Exercises

Acknowledgements

Lynne

For their professional advice and support, I would like to thank Piers Chandler and Sally Gardner. I am also indebted to the staff at The Beadle House Sports Injury Clinic, in particular to Sarah Ashwell and Susan Kortum.

Working with Helge has been great fun, and immensely rewarding.

My clients in Sevenoaks continue to inspire me and I am very grateful for their continuing patience and support.

As life gets more hectic, the importance of having an understanding, supportive family becomes very apparent. I cannot thank enough my daughters, Rebecca and Emily, and also my parents-in-law, Stella and Vic. My own parents died before the publication of my first book and therefore knew nothing of my new-found career. However, I am acutely aware that, without their loving care, none of this would have been possible.

Helge

Writing a book had never really crossed my mind until I met Lynne. I thank her for the trust she has put in me and for the very enjoyable co-writing.

I would like to thank Anja Dashwood for all the inspiration and friendship over the years and, especially, Paul for supporting me during the very busy times.

Lynne and I would like to thank Gordon Thomson for his friendship, advice and stimulating ideas.

Finally, we would like to mention a very special person who has helped us in so many ways. Leigh has often worked through the night to meet the deadlines and has always been there for us both.

A special thank you to Lesley Howling, the photographer, not just for her wonderful photographic skills but also for feeding us so well!

We must also thank our models:
Sarah Hatchuel
David Bargeron, I.T. consultant.
Victor Robinson, grandfather and retired security consultant.

Foreword by Gordon Thomson

Lynne Robinson

I didn't quite know what I had let myself in for when I agreed to train Lynne in the Pilates Method! Although she had good experience in the Method from her time in Sydney, Australia, she wasn't a dancer and she had no background in fitness at all. Furthermore, she had a history of back and neck problems. What struck me instantly, though, was her single-mindedness and determination. She worked hard on her own body and then researched in depth so that she fully understood what the exercises and the technique were doing and why.

Lynne had been a history teacher before her travels abroad and, so, teaching came naturally to her. This academic background enabled her to take a completely different approach to Pilates. She wanted it studied and explained. On top of this, her own injuries and her lack of experience in movement teaching meant that she was coming to the exercises as a lay person — this has given her a very special empathy with people who have back problems. She knows what it's like to start exercising from scratch and, as a result, has simplified and clarified the classical Pilates matwork exercises, breaking them down in such a way that they are easily understood and followed by everyone.

The writing and the launch of our first book together *Body Control: The Pilates Way* in March 1997, was a milestone in both our lives. Neither of us could have envisaged that it would so quickly become a bestseller. The runaway success of that first book also led to the demand for Pilates teachers increasing a hundredfold, in anticipation of which the Body Control Pilates Teacher Training partnership was formed by Lynne, Helge and myself. It has proved a resounding success and, hopefully, will be a key factor in realizing our joint ambition that, within the near future, Pilates becomes accessible to all.

Helge Fisher

If Lynne is a natural teacher, then Helge is a natural liberator! It was during a Pilates mat class at the London Studio Centre in 1986 that I first noticed her unique talent. Helge's own body has innate grace and freedom of movement. She is not selfish with her gift; sharing it by helping others to attain the same freedom – she, quite literally, liberates bodies.

It was a natural step for her to train with me in the Pilates Method and having taught Pilates for 13 years, she has recently set up her own studio in Brighton, Sussex. Her thirst for knowledge led her to develop her training further by following a three-year course in the Alexander Technique and by gaining an ITEC certificate in massage, which she now teaches in addition to her Pilates teacher training work.

'Teaching movement is seeing, as teaching music is hearing', said Pilates master Eve Gentry. Well, if this is the case, Helge has 20:20 vision! She can spot a client's misalignment or any source of tension from the other side of the room and, as you watch her work to release that tension and realign the body, you are left in no doubt that here is a body worker of the highest calibre.

I am delighted that Lynne and Helge have come together to write this book and I know that 'bodies' everywhere will benefit and will share in my enthusiasm.

'From the moment we wake up, we spend the entire day hunched over a desk, a steering wheel, a cooker, the baby or even a surgical table! It is wonderful to have found a method of exercise to reverse this, to help us uncoil, to length and 'iron us' out.

That this exercise is also both relaxing and enjoyable adds to its attraction. As a practising GP, I know that so many of my patients would benefit enormously from the exercises within this book.'

Richard Husband MB, Ch.B., DRCOG

'I feel, as a practitioner, that this book is vital to support and strengthen patients' recovery and well being. F. Alexander and Joseph Pilates were pioneers in body use and, as a consequence, general health. The Mind Body Workout is essential for health and illustrates techniques for everyone to use – the section on Basic Rules for Good Body Use is especially relevant to everyday life.

I can only recommend this book wholeheartedly.'

Timothy John, DO MRO, Registered Osteopath

What Can This Book Do For You?

This is much more than just a book about exercise. It will change the way you move, the way you feel, the way you think and, last but not least, the way you look!

We believe we are all entitled to bodies that work. The simple directions laid out in the following pages can help you restore and maintain the natural health and balance of your body.

Not only will you look terrific (the conditioning exercises will reshape and realign you), but you will feel different too – this is a workout designed to liberate both mind and body.

Introduction

'It is the mind itself that builds the body' Schiller

Though different in character and background, F. M. Alexander and Joseph Pilates, nevertheless, had much in common. Both had physical shortcomings which they refused to accept and both, as a result, worked on their own bodies, experimenting until they found methods which helped them overcome their specific weaknesses. Rather than accepting already established systems to improve their bodies, they continued, until the last, to explore their own potential from within. Others saw the changes and asked to be instructed in the techniques that they developed – and so, we now have the legacy that they have left to us: simple directions for good body use. We would like you to follow in their footsteps by exploring your own bodies, allowing us to offer you guidelines and, perhaps, to open some new dimensions. As you progress you should ultimately be listening less and less to our directions and increasingly to your own bodies, to what some may call your 'inner wisdom'. We want to reintroduce you to yourself, inviting you to take a fresh

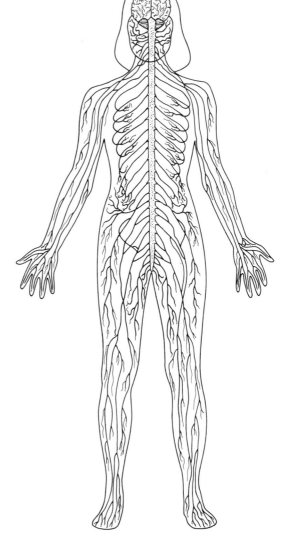

The Pathways of the Nervous System

approach to how you use your body in daily life and exercise and to rediscover the pathways from your mind to your body. These neurological pathways may not be functioning efficiently because, quite simply, they have not been trodden for a while so, as a result, they have become overgrown like a path in a jungle.

Only by using these pathways again and again, do we learn to recognize them easily. . .

What is Wrong with the Way we Use
Our Bodies?

The Lost World of the Senses

It's like living on a diet of mashed potato! Our lives are so comfortable, so bland, that many of us have now lost the ability to 'read' our senses. They have been numbed by our sheltered existence and, as our survival no longer depends on them, we have come to disregard them.

Where is the raw excitement or, indeed, the danger that our forebears had to face? When were you last chased by a hairy mammoth? Today, we seek these kind of 'thrills' by going to disaster movies, by taking the most spectacular ride in a theme park, by going white-water rafting or bungee jumping. It is really not surprising how popular these diversions have become because the sheer physical 'buzz' we experience during them is essentially a substitute for the real challenges that our ancestors once faced.

When the adrenaline is pumping we know we are alive. For most of the time, however, we are back to the 'mashed potato' and our way of life is just not challenging enough to keep us mentally and physically fit. Constantly being 'kept' at the right temperature, fed well before we are hungry,

sleeping at a preordained hour rather than because we are tired, our bodies are even tricked into believing it is day when it is night, and vice-versa – our natural biofeedback system is confused. A couple of weeks in a five-star hotel may be wonderfully relaxing, but aren't our senses dulled by the blandness of it all?

We were once forced to live, and survive, by those senses. We relied on them to tell us if there was danger and to respond – if we were thirsty to find water, if hungry to hunt food. Today's environmentally 'controlled' existence means that we have lost the instinctive responses of our bodies. Or rather, they are still there but we have forgotten how to interpret them and react to them appropriately.

You will be pleased to know that we are not suggesting that you all sign up for the nearest sky diving course! We do, however, need to waken up the senses. In order to develop good body use you must learn to sense with fresh feeling. Aristotle handed down to us the tradition of the five senses of touch, taste, smell, sight and hearing. These senses inform us about the world around us and are relevant to good body use. But, of equal importance is the 'kinaesthetic' sense, which Aristotle omitted.

This sense informs us not about the external world but, rather, the internal, our inner world. Our kinaesthetic awareness is an awareness of how we use our bodies and, as most of us in the western world have lost this sense, we are quite literally out of touch with our bodies.

Stress

'Complete freedom from stress is death'

H. Seyle

Modern medicine may have won in its battles against its old enemies – the epidemics of infectious diseases – but new enemies have since emerged. Many of the major killers today like cancer and heart disease are known to be stress-related. Are our lives so much more stressful than our ancestors'? They had hunger, thirst, cold and sheer survival to cope with, we have unemployment, moving, divorce and the mortgage. Not all stress is harmful. It is integral to life itself. Without it, we would never be spurred on or challenged. Indeed, it is not the stress itself which harms us but rather the we way we respond to it and, in particular, how we return our bodies to normal following stress; how we unwind. There's the problem, for many of us do not seem to be able to escape from stress in the same way that our ancestors did. Although not life threatening, our modern day 'mam-

moths' are more complicated to solve. In many ways it was easier to deal with the immediate danger of being trampled or eaten alive – you were confronted with two choices: stay and fight or run like mad! We may well be tempted to react in the same way with the final demand bill from the electricity or gas company, but, in reality, this stress will probably take longer to go away.

As a result, our bodies remain ready for action, in 'fight or flight' mode, which means that many of our basic bodily functions, those not vital to the task of battle, stay shut down. Unfortunately, this includes our immune system – our natural self-repair system. Technically, it is the parasympathetic part of the autonomic nervous system which regulates the 'let down' from stress and re-establishes self-repair. Anti-inflammatory or anti-stress hormones are released into the blood. Learning to relax and release tension is vital to both this counterbalance to stress and, generally, to good body use. As both the mind and the body are involved in the process, we must re-educate both.

Are you Sitting Comfortably?

We hope not! Well, not for too long anyway.

For most of the time we slump in chairs that are poorly designed, but even 'ergonomically designed' chairs can add to our postural problems by encouraging us to sit for longer when we really should be moving about. Just try adding up how many hours of the day you spend sitting in the home, the office, the car, the bus. It really is quite frightening! This sedentary lifestyle with its lack of variety of movement has thrown our whole muscular system totally out of balance (see page 24). We simply do not move enough.

Off to the Gym

There is no doubt that we are now far more fitness conscious than ever, as is clearly demonstrated by the growth in fitness and leisure centres. Unfortunately, there is a similar growth in the number of sports injury clinics! The increase in the number of fitness-related injuries is a reliable indicator that whilst we may be exercising more, many of us are also harming ourselves in the process. Why?

Part of the problem is that we are not fit to undertake our fitness routine! How many of us, for our New Year's resolution, signed up for the local fitness class, only to drop out because we felt worse after it than before? How many middle-aged 'born again' footballers end up on the injury bench before half-time?

The problem is that we have lost the ability to use our bodies well, so we continue to stress our bodies during the exercise itself by still more misuse. Whether you go to the gym, to aerobics, to yoga, whether you play a team or competitive sport, if you do not use your body well during any exer-

cise, you will harm yourself. Even professional athletes, sportsmen and dancers punish their bodies during the prime of their careers and frequently pay a high price for it later in life.

Good Body Use = Mind Body Work

The aim of this book, therefore, is to introduce you to good body use through Mind Body work. This 'good use' should be continued into your daily activities as well as your exercise routines. We hope to re-educate your body and introduce sound movement patterns which you can use whatever your profession, whatever your chosen sport or fitness regime. The lessons learnt here will benefit the ballet dancer and the rugby player, the first-time exerciser or the athlete.

To do this, to reconnect our mind, body and senses, we have to work on the neurological pathways that connect the mind to the muscles. These neurological pathways form the nervous system which co-ordinates all our movements. Some of these movements are under our voluntary control whilst others are automatic – imagine the hassles involved if we had to be conscious of the process involved with breathing. Our conscious control is limited to starting and stopping, and to the direction, range, speed and force of our movements. So, we decide what we want to do, give the go-ahead and we then let the nervous system select the choice of muscles whose co-ordinated work

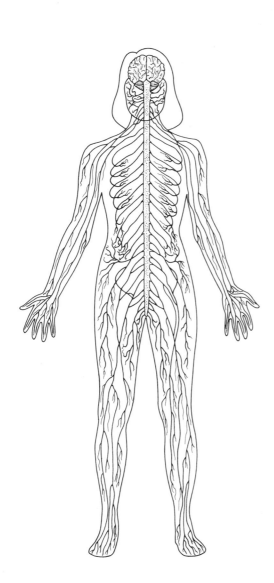

The Pathways of the Nervous System

will achieve that goal, and choose the nerve pathways over which the messages will travel. This is where good and bad body use step in, where habit and habitual misuse, where existing muscle imbalances can cause harm. Established habits are difficult to change but it is possible, through relinking and co-ordinating the neuromuscular pathways, for the habitual balance and movement patterns to be re-educated.

'My body was always just something that carried my head around,' remarked one client. We hope that with the new approach to exercise laid out in this book, we will put the body and mind back together into a good working relationship. You will need to be constantly and consciously aware of the movements of the exercises, what they feel like, where you are working, whether there is tension elsewhere.

To do this we have to redevelop your body awareness, to reawaken the senses and then re-train the body in its movement patterns so that you can act appropriately. In this way the body will become highly tuned. Energy is no longer being wasted unnecessarily but, rather, being used effectively. With the balance restored, the in-built capacity of our bodies for self-healing is given a chance.

Two Men, Two Methods

F. M. Alexander (1869–1955) and his Technique

The Alexander Technique takes its name from an Australian actor, F. M. Alexander, born in 1869. His career was threatened by his persistent throat problems, which frequently led to a temporary loss of voice. As doctors failed to help him on numerous occasions, Alexander embarked on a unique journey of self-discovery to find a cure for his problem.

He decided to observe himself in the mirror to see if he could find out whether any particular actions or mannerisms during reciting (which was very fashionable at that time) caused his vocal problem. After several months, Alexander discovered that he, in fact, stiffened his neck and pulled his head back and down. On further observation he also noticed that this way of using his voice was part of a muscular tension pattern, which included how he used his own body. This pattern influenced everything he did, and he noticed changes of the balance-poise of his head, neck and back. He came to the conclusion that changing the way he used these parts was

the key to improving the general use of his body.

Furthermore, Alexander discovered that this faulty pattern also occurred at the moment he got ready to recite! The thought of a movement or activity alone was enough to 'trigger' his pattern, almost like a reflex. He had to learn to stop himself doing this before he started reciting to reaffirm his new way of using his head, neck and back – this can also be called active non-doing (see Release the chapter on relaxation). As a result of these discoveries, Alexander's voice improved and he experienced much greater freedom of movement in general.

In 1904, he moved to London where he soon built a flourishing practice working with many people from the theatre, his students including Sir Henry Shaw, Lily Langtry, George Bernard Shaw and Aldous Huxley. From there it was but a small step to start training other teachers, which he did from 1913 through to his death in 1955 with the result that, today, there are training courses held throughout the world.

People often associate the Alexander Technique solely with 'posture'. This word suggests something static and yet a teacher of the Alexander Technique is actually more interested and concerned with movement in the body.

With the help of a teacher (or by following the explorations in this book over a period of time) you will become more aware of faulty patterns of body use that have replaced your natural ease of movement. The Technique helps to give more attention to *how* you perform even the simplest of daily tasks and is less concerned with specific movements (although certain suggestions will be made). Gradually your body will become a more sensitive 'instrument', enabling you to move with less strain and waste of energy.

There are some basic principles to the Alexander Technique

▷ Recognizing the 'use' of the body with its harmful patterns.
▷ Learning how to stop in order to allow change to happen and to 'undo' the knots.
▷ Re-educating the kinaesthetic sense.
▷ Quieting the mind to focus on the mind–body connection.
▷ Establishing a good head–neck relationship.

Some of these principles will be explained in detail in the opening chapters.

Observing your body use

As you read this book, pause for a moment and give attention to the position you are in:

▷ Is your back straight or bent?
▷ What is happening in your shoulders?
▷ Is your head to one side?
▷ What position are your legs in?
▷ Are your feet touching the floor?
▷ Where are your arms?
▷ What expression is on your face?
▷ How long have you been in this position?
▷ Do you notice any stiffness or discomfort in your body?
▷ Do you notice any other sensations in your body?

These are all observations about how you are using yourself while reading. Try not do judge what you are doing, just observe.

The way we do things in our daily life is central to the Alexander Technique, for Alexander discovered a way to continually improve our body use in all that we do. Everything can either be done in a good way that promotes healthy functioning or in a way that is harmful to our functioning, with many of these negative habits being very common indeed.

Habitual behaviour is something we do without having consciously to think about it, allowing our minds to give attention to other things – for example, as a child you had to learn to stand, yet, as an adult, you can easily wash the dishes while standing! Our behaviour becomes more complex. This is fine, if we learned our skills in a way that is beneficial to us. It only creates a problem when we find problems and want to change the way we are doing things. In order to change, we have once again to start consciously thinking about how we are doing something. It can be very difficult to undo habitual behaviour and learning precisely how to do this is a large part of the Alexander Technique.

Quieting the mind

Thoughts, images and inner dialogue will be coming and going, especially when you try to concentrate during the following exercises and explorations. To be honest, you will probably be even more aware of them than usual which, in itself, is an important part of Mind Body awareness. Do not worry that your mind is constantly moving – observe whatever happens and let it pass naturally. It will gradually become easier to focus on internal processes and those unwanted thoughts about our everyday problems will pass more quickly.

The Head–Neck Relationship

One of the most fundamental discoveries that Alexander made was the importance of the head–neck relationship.

The typical weight of the head is about five to six kilos. A very heavy part of us! This heavy head balances on top of the spine in such a way that the centre of gravity of the head is forward of the point of pivot of the skull. The head is prevented from falling forward all the time by muscles which con-

nect the back of the skull to other parts of the skeleton. Watch someone falling asleep in a sitting position and you can observe how the head falls forward as these muscles release – they have truly 'nodded off'. When we are awake, however, we are not aware of these muscles working to keep the head upright; this is automatic or habitual to our waking state. Alexander discovered that there is a tendency in human beings to 'pull the head back', as a result of which these muscles shorten, often chronically.

The 'Startle Reflex' is a response of the body which occurs in response to stress or shock. Initially muscles of the head and neck tighten and shorten, pulling the head back and down. From there, the tension 'spreads', resulting in raised shoulders and stiffened arms. Whenever there is a sudden noise like the slamming of a door or the backfire of a car, we react in this way out of pure reflex and, naturally, the greater the stress we are under, the more likely this is to happen. As a result of this 'Startle Reflex' we not only pull our heads back and down but compress our spine at the same time. This creates a shortening and narrowing of the back.

Alexander was of the opinion that in undoing these problems we begin to allow the sub-occipital muscles to do their work of balancing the head on the spine – the semi supine position on page 46 is a good start to reversing this process. To counteract this 'back and down' pull, Alexander decided that the head needed to be released forward and up, as shown in the illustration on page 21.

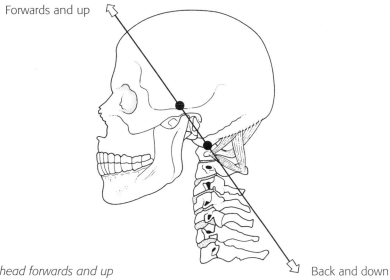

Forwards and up

Back and down

Release your head forwards and up

This, in turn, stimulates all the releasing mechanisms in the body so that, as a result, the body moves in a co-ordinated and integrated way with the head leading the movement. In all vertebrates the head acts as the organizer of movement. This can be observed particularly in four-legged animals, like cats, who follow their senses with the body organizing its movement around the initial movement of the head.

Alexander named this head–neck relationship 'Primary Control'. When it is functioning well it gives rise to the greatest ease of movement, allowing the head to balance freely on the spine.

Throughout this book we will be suggesting that you should 'stand tall', lengthening your back. This is can be achieved much more easily if you release the neck muscles and carry your head with the minimal amount of tension.

Joseph Pilates (1880–1967) and his Method

Like Alexander, Joseph Pilates had to overcome a physical weakness. Born in 1880 in Düsseldorf, he was a frail sickly child, but was determined to overcome this fragility. Instead of following an established fitness regime, he experimented with many different approaches and one can, in fact, recognize the different elements of these methods in his own teaching. Yoga, gymnastics, skiing, self-defence, dance, circus training and weight training all influenced him and he chose aspects of each to develop his own body. By absorbing these other methods, selecting the most effective aspects from each, Joseph was able to work out a system which had the perfect balance of strength and flexibility.

Proven on his own body, he then began

to apply these techniques to others. When living in Britain at the time of the First World War, he was interned because of his nationality. With time on his hands, he developed his technique and began to train his fellow internees with amazing success. Later, when he moved to the United States of America and set up a studio with his wife Clara in New York in the 1920s, he soon attracted top ballet dancers, actors and actresses, gymnasts and athletes, all anxious to learn from him.

Unlike Alexander, however, Joseph never took the initiative of setting up an official training programme with the result that many of his disciples went on to teach their own versions of Pilates Method. The definition of what was, or is, true Pilates is somewhat blurred and, indeed, is still being debated today. It is not helped by the fact that Joseph rarely taught the same exercise in the same way two days running, partly because he geared his teaching to the needs of the individual, teaching a completely different set of exercises to each client. Some of these clients themselves went on to teach, each one therefore working with a different emphasis.

Pilates has now been taught for over seventy years and yet it is only in the last few years that the medical profession has really begun to look closely at why the system is so successful. Until then, many Pilates teachers taught intuitively, learning during apprenticeship about good alignment and good body use, but, in many cases, without fully knowing the technical medical framework for what they were doing. Under the close scrutiny of the medical world, we have had to re-examine our methods and study precisely why they work so well.

There is a common philosophy at the root of all Pilates-based methods, stemming from the manner in which one approaches the exercises – it is less about *what* you do, more about *how* you do it! This has been a great advantage to Pilates teachers as they have been able to absorb new ideas – for example in physiotherapy techniques or movement therapies – and incorporate them into the Method without sacrificing its uniqueness. As a result, Pilates continues to evolve as a system, to move forward without the constraint of a rigid set of rules.

Body Control Pilates is just one of the systems to evolve from the work of Joseph Pilates. It is a version of the Pilates Method developed by Gordon Thomson, a teacher of twenty-one years' standing, and Lynne Robinson. It is characterized by the 'Eight Principles' which are applied to each and every exercise:

▷ Relaxation
▷ Concentration
▷ Alignment
▷ Centring
▷ Breathing
▷ Co-ordination
▷ Flowing Movements
▷ Stamina

Briefly, the Method works by initially teaching you how to relax and release unnecessary tension from the body. You are taught to focus your attention on the body, increasing your level of awareness so that you are familiar with good and bad alignment. You are trained to breathe correctly and to time the breath with movement to best advantage. Learning to isolate and use your deep abdominal muscles to support the spine for each and every movement you make is crucial to the programme and is one of the many reasons why Pilates is so effective in helping people who have back problems. Once you have learnt to stabilize your torso, we add small movements while you maintain this 'core stability'. We then build on to this slowly, adding stretching and strengthening exercises to rebalance the body, but always with the strong centre. Finally, you have to co-ordinate all this – the alignment, the breathing, the centring and in so doing sound movement patterns are introduced. The advanced exercises are choreographed so that they are very challenging, even for the professional athlete or dancer. Moving always with slow flowing movements, the exercises look deceptively easy, but most people often do not realize that it is harder to do an exercise slowly than it is to rush it. By working in this way, you cannot cheat and the strength that is built into the body gives great endurance and stamina. Although it is not an aerobic exercise programme as such, when you reach the advanced levels the exercises can be performed aerobically if you want to. For most of us however, we recommend that you add some brisk walking or swimming into your schedule.

Why is Pilates different from other fitness regimes?

This is a difficult question to answer but the best way is to use a simple simile. Body Control Pilates works on the deep architectural structure of the body by targeting the key postural muscles, so that we literally work from the inside out. Compare the body to a house – for many of us the building is in urgent need of repair! Perhaps the roof tiles are falling off, cracks appearing in the plaster, paint peeling. There may even be electrical and plumbing faults! These are often just signs indicating more serious structural problems. You can call in the plasterers or the decorators but, in a few months' time, the same problems will reappear unless you tackle the underlying faults.

Many fitness regimes are concerned only with the superficial, cosmetic aspects of exercise, the 'hips, bums and tums' approach. Pilates works deeper, building strength from the inside. We are, in fact, far more effective at achieving the flat stomach, trim thighs and well-rounded bottom that, let's be honest, we all want – but we get these results safely and they last! The Pilates teacher is effectively the 'structural engineer' for the body. The exercises are designed to correct misalignments and to provide structural support for the body. We tackle the foundations of the building and put in the necessary supporting beams! So, we build strength from the inside out, realign the body and thus restore the balance.

We talk a great deal about muscle imbalance and sound movement pattern, but what exactly do we mean? We have already mentioned the sedentary lifestyle of modern man. Let us, for a moment, take a simplified view and study the muscle imbalances of the average person.

Sitting hunched over a desk all day, the muscles of the chest around the front of the shoulders (the pectoral muscles) become excessively tight. Add to this the way in which we all tense our shoulders up to our ears and tip our head back when stressed – 'the Startle Reflex' – and you have the muscles of the upper shoulders and neck – the upper trapezius, levator scapulae and sternocleidomastoid – all over-worked. Meanwhile, the muscles of the mid-back, in particular those which stabilize the shoulder blades – the lower trapezius, the rhomboids, serratus anterior, the teres and latissimus dorsi – may become over-stretched, over-lengthened and weak.

Sitting for long periods means that the muscles that normally bend the knee on the trunk (the hip flexors) are overused and become short and tight. Meanwhile, the lower abdominals and the buttocks (the gluteals) are weak and the hamstrings short. The low back itself is usually stiff and immobile. Basically, for most of us, the

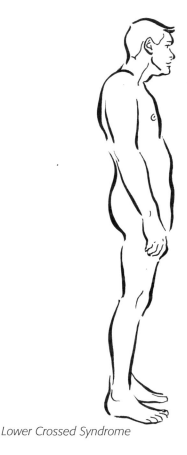

Lower Crossed Syndrome

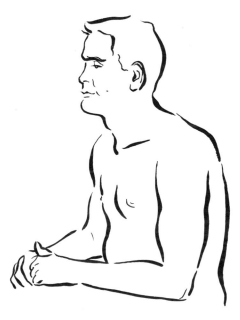

Upper Crossed Syndrome

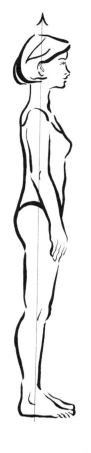

The mid-back, scapular stabilizing muscles, muscles need strengthening.

The upper body needs 'opening', the pectorals stretching.

The buttocks (gluteals) need strengthening.

The abdominals need strengthening.

The hamstrings usually need stretching.

The hip flexors need stretching.

Correcting the imbalances –
Side-on view

following needs to happen (see diagram).

Once you start to work on correcting these muscle imbalances, the body becomes more balanced. But what about movement patterns? Muscles work in groups to produce movement. If one of the muscles in a group is too tight or too weak, the whole movement pattern is upset, the muscle group cannot do its job properly. But we still want to move, so the body cheats and uses other muscles to do the work, effectively sending in the substitutes. This substitution creates a bad movement pattern. This is the 'habitual misuse' of the Alexander Technique.

In order to correct the problem, we have first to release and lengthen the tight muscles, then strengthen the weak ones and, thereafter, teach the body the right muscles combinations, the sound movement patterns.

This is what Pilates exercises are all about, this is why over the last seventy years Pilates has succeeded in helping not only professionals to achieve their maximum performance potential, but also to rehabilitate people with severe injuries. And – we do it in an interesting and challenging way. There is nothing more tedious than 'remedial exercises'! 'Science meets the Arts' in Pilates – the exercises are creative, but also medically-sound and approved.

A Fresh New Approach to
Body Use and Exercise

Both Pilates and the Alexander Technique are Mind Body methods which concern themselves with good body use. Both require you to be sensitive to what is happening in your body, to be thoughtful of your movements. Neither technique has any religious basis at all and are equally suitable within 'mainstream' or 'complementary' medical practice. You are free to follow your own conscience. However, we do believe that good body use has no disciplinary boundaries and therefore we have also discussed and drawn on some other techniques as well, such as massage techniques, yoga, Chi Kung, T'ai Chi, Feldenkrais and the Mezières Method.

Let's now introduce you to what we have called the 'Building Blocks' of this Mind Body Workout:

▷ Release
▷ Awareness
▷ Breathing
▷ Use of centre
▷ Grounding
▷ Balance
▷ Directing – Pathways

In all of the chapters, we will be looking at a different aspect of body use with each containing a selection of 'explorations' and exercises. The idea behind these explorations is that you learn how to experience and sense yourself in new ways in relation to space, the ground and the objects around you, like taking a leisurely journey inside and around yourself.

The exercises are all from the Body Control Pilates Method. In order to practice them safely, it is very important that you read and try the basic exercises in the chapter covering 'Basic Rules'. With these on board, you can then proceed with confidence. The exercises do vary in difficulty, but we have clearly indicated when they are advanced.

At first, you will find that you can only accomplish one thing at a time. While you concentrate on your breathing, your 'navel to spine' may slip, but, just as when you first learned to drive and could only manage the steering and braking whilst the gears were impossible to fathom, you will soon be able to co-ordinate easily all the aspects of all the building blocks. You will then be well on your way to the ultimate Mind Body Workout.

So, before you begin:

▷ Be sure that you have no pressing unfinished business.
▷ Take the telephone off the hook, or put the answering machine on.
▷ You may prefer silence, otherwise put on some unobtrusive classical or new age music.
▷ All exercises should be done on a padded mat.
▷ Wear something warm and comfortable, allowing free movement.
▷ Barefoot is best, socks otherwise.

The best time to exercise is in the late afternoon or evening when your muscles are already warmed up as a result of the day's activity. Exercising in the morning is fine, but you will need to take longer to warm up thoroughly.

You will need space to work in – you cannot keep stopping to move furniture. Some clear wall space is also useful.

Items you may need include a chair, a small flat but firm pillow for behind your head or perhaps a folded towel, a larger pillow, a long scarf and a tennis ball.

Please do not exercise if:

▷ You are feeling unwell.
▷ You have just eaten a heavy meal.
▷ You have been drinking alcohol.
▷ You are in pain from an injury – always consult your practitioner first, as rest may be needed before you exercise.

▷ You have taken pain killers, as it will mask any warning pains.
▷ You are undergoing medical treatment, or are taking drugs – again, you will need to consult your medical practitioner first.
▷ And remember, it is always wise to consult your doctor before taking up a new exercise regime.

Not all of the exercises are suitable for use during pregnancy. However, you may like to try the special session at the back of the book.

If you have a back problem you will need to consult with your medical practitioner. Many of the exercises are wonderful for back-related problems but you will need expert guidance. We have put together a special session to help with back trouble at the end of the book.

Getting Started

To give you a clear picture of the goals of the Mind Body Workout, we suggest that you start off by reading through the first few introductory chapters, then read the opening pages to each of the Seven Building Blocks. At the end, we have outlined sessions which form balanced workouts. Ideally, you should aim to do at least three of these a week – although daily would be wonderful!

As a taster of how the explorations and exercises actually work, read through the following basic rules for good body use, then try the following:

▷ Relaxation Position (page 46).
▷ Use of Centre – Co-ordinating Arms and Legs (page 120).
▷ Side Rolls (page 124).
▷ Standing Like a Tree (page 134).
▷ Beach Ball Hamstrings (page 94).
▷ Pillow Squeeze (page 82).
▷ Chalk Circle (page 122).
▷ Melting Body (page 92).

As you become more familiar with the explorations and exercises, you will want to devise your own programmes. Just bear in mind that you need to balance front, back and sideways movements, strength and flexibility, and relaxing and stimulating exercises.

But above all, have fun!

Some Basic Rules to
Good Body Use in Exercise

Before you can attempt any of the exercises in this book, there are certain fundamentals of sound body use that you need to understand and learn.

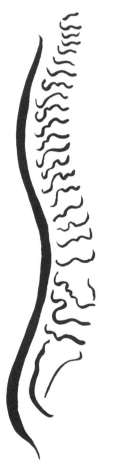

Spine curves

The Neutral Position of the Pelvis and Spine

What do we mean by 'neutral' and why is it so important? If you look at the shape of the spine, you will see that it is an 'S' shape with natural curves.

These curves develop during early childhood and enable the spine to absorb some of the shock which would otherwise be transmitted up to our head when we move. The postural muscles of the body are, as we stand, working constantly to keep us upright. There exists a delicate balance between those at the front of the body and those at the back, and any habitual change in the way we stand or sit will affect that balance. The spinal ligaments are affected in a similar way. If you repeatedly bend forwards or backwards, the ligaments will lengthen and the balance is upset. Furthermore, the pressure within the spinal discs will increase. Sitting slumped over your desk all day alters the angles of the curves of the spine and stresses these ligaments, muscles and discs. Eventually, pain can set in.

If you then exercise without due attention to your postural alignment, you are just adding fuel to the fire. So, you must have your spine in its natural neutral position when you exercise.

The pelvis is connected to the spine. It is balanced on the hip joints and can tilt one way or the other, pulling the lumbar spine with it, which will again stress those spinal tissues. A natural neutral position is needed to maintain the tissues at their normal length, and keep the disc pressure low.

That's the theory, so how about the practice? It is one thing paying lip service to the neutral pelvis and spine position, but you must absolutely learn to recognize it for yourself if you are to exercise correctly and safely. For this, you need improved body awareness through which you have to be able to detect even small variations in the angle of the pelvis.

We recommend that you check your pelvic/spine angle constantly while you are doing the exercises. Meanwhile, the following routine will help you to find and identify neutral. To find your natural, neutral pelvis and spine position, try the following:

Finding Neutral

Lie on your back with your knees bent and feet hip width apart and in parallel. Imagine that you have a compass on your lower abdomen, the navel is North, the pubic bone South, with West and East on either side.

We are going to look at two incorrect

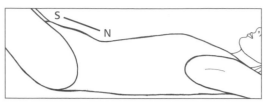

Tilted to North

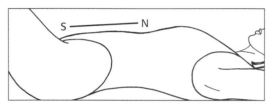

Tilted to South

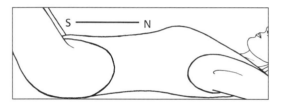

Neutral – the correct natural position of the pelvis

positions in order to find the correct one. Tilt your pelvis up toward North – while doing so, the pelvis will 'tuck under'. Notice what has happened to your waist, your hips and your tailbone (which is at the top of the crease of your buttocks). The waist is flattened, you've pushed it into the floor, the curve is lost. You have gripped the muscles around your hips and your tailbone has lifted off the floor.

Now, carefully (avoid this bit if you have a back injury), bring the pelvis so that it is tilting towards South. Now notice again what has happened. The low back is arched and feels vulnerable, your ribs have flared, you probably have two chins and your stomach is sticking out.

We are aiming for a neutral position between the two extremes, neither to North nor South, neither tucked nor arched. Back with the image of the compass, the pointer is level like a spirit level. The tailbone remains down on floor and lengthens away. The pelvis keeps its length and is not 'scrunched up' at all.

There remains a small natural arch in your back. This is neutral, and all the exercises should be performed in this neutral position unless you are told otherwise. You would not start your car if the gears were not in neutral, so please do not start an exercise without being in the correct position! Be particularly vigilant when you are engaging the lower abdominals (see page 34), as there is a temptation to tilt or tuck the pelvis. If you are lying down, you can always try placing your hand under your waist – you will feel then if you are pushing the spine into the floor. You want to avoid this.

It is also worth pointing out that if you have a large bottom, you will have more of a hollow in the lumbar region. This does not necessarily mean that you have arched your back. Learn to recognize your natural curve.

Breathing

The next fundamental is correct breathing. In order for the body to receive enough oxygen to perform the exercises, we must breathe efficiently and deeply. However, ask most people to breathe deeply and they will do one of two things: they will raise their shoulders up around their ears and arch their back or, alternatively, they will breathe deep into their lower abdominals. The first is too shallow, while the second is great for relaxation and yoga but impossible for Pilates, where we need to keep those lower abdominals back to the spine (see page 34)! That leaves us only one way to go – wide. This makes sound sense as our lungs are situated in the ribcage, so, by expanding the ribcage, the volume of the cavity is increased and therefore the capacity for oxygen intake is increased. This type of breathing also works the muscles between the ribs, encouraging their expansion and it helps to make the upper body more fluid and mobile.

We call it thoracic or lateral breathing. Your lungs become like bellows, the lower ribcage expanding wide as you breathe in and closing down as you breathe out. We do not wish to block the descent of the diaphragm but, rather, we encourage the movement to be widthways and into the back.

Scarf breathing

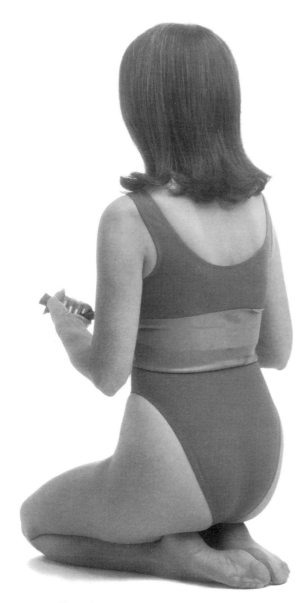

Scarf breathing

To practice try the following:

Sit or stand and wrap a scarf or towel around your ribs, crossing it over at the front.

Holding the opposite ends of the scarf and pulling it gently tight, breathe in and allow your ribs to expand the scarf. As you breathe out, you may gently squeeze the scarf to help you fully empty your lungs and relax the ribcage, allowing the breastbone to soften. Just watch that you do not lift the breastbone too high.

Not only is the type of breathing important to our way of exercising, but also the timing of the breath. You can help or hinder a movement by breathing in or out. All Pilates exercises are designed carefully to reinforce and encourage the correct right muscle recruitment by using the breath. Most people find this timing difficult at first, especially if you are used to other fitness regimes, but once you have mastered it, it makes sense. As a general rule, we:

▷ Breathe in to prepare for a movement
▷ Breathe out, navel to spine, and move
▷ Breathe in to recover

Moving on the exhalation will enable you to relax into the stretch and prevent you from tensing up. It also safeguards against you holding your breath, which can unduly stress the heart and lead to serious complications.

Navel to Spine

It was over seventy-five years ago that Joseph Pilates first discovered the importance of drawing the navel back to the spine for each movement. He was well ahead of his time on this and had, in fact, discovered what the medical profession now refers to as 'core stability'.

Muscles have several roles to play in

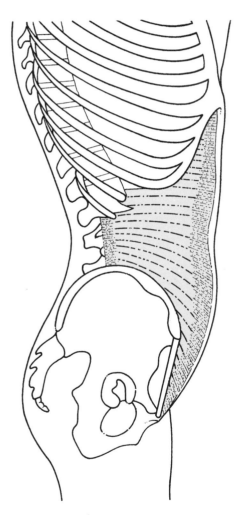

Transversus muscle

movement and, of course, without them we would not be going anywhere. They move our limbs but our trunk has to remain stable, otherwise we would fall over when we raised a leg or an arm, for example. In Pilates we are equally, if not more, concerned with the muscles that keep your torso stable as we are with the moving limbs. These muscles lie deep within the body and work to make the trunk into a more solid cylinder, so that we have a solid base for our arms and legs to push against.

The muscles to which we are referring are the tranversus abdominis, the internal obliques (and the multifidus – part of the back stabilizing group). Unfortunately, they are not worked during the exercises of standard fitness regimes, where the commonly practised 'sit ups' tend to work the rectus abdominis instead, at the expense of the deeper muscles. The Pilates Method has always concentrated instead on the deeper core muscles. You can feel them easily for yourself by simply placing your hands around your waist and coughing – those are the muscles we are talking about.

We try to teach you how to identify and isolate the key muscles. Then, you learn to engage them sufficiently so that they support the spine, which means using them at about forty per cent of their capability. As postural muscles they need endurance training rather than speed or strength training, so forty per cent is about right as a usage figure, especially as you must remember that during the course of an hour's exercise you can be engaging them hundreds of times. When you have found the right muscles and can engage them properly, we then make life harder by adding on movements. In daily life you are moving around so these muscles have to be able to function while you perform daily tasks. Slowly, we start to add more complicated movements, some of them quite choreographed.

The trunk must stay stable while you perform these movements. An exercise like Scissors on page 176 requires 'core stability' if it is to be done with no harm to your back.

So this is what we are aiming for, but let's now go right back to the beginning. First we have to find the right muscles.

▷ Lie on your back. Check that your pelvis is in neutral.
▷ Breathe in to prepare. Lengthen up through the top of your head.
▷ Breathe out and draw the lower abdominals back towards the spine, hollowing out your lower stomach. *Do not allow the pelvis to tuck under*. Do not

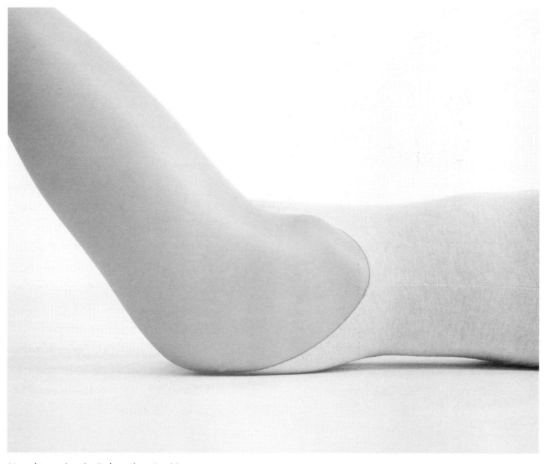

Navel to spine in Relaxation Position

push into the spine. Keep your tailbone on the floor and lengthening away.

▷ Breathe in and relax.

You must be careful not to tuck the pelvis under, that is tilting it to North. If you do, you will lose your neutral position (see page 30) and it means that other muscles – the rectus abdominis and the hip flexors – are doing the work instead of the tranversus and internal obliques. If you are comfortable with your hand under your waist you can check to see if you are pushing into the spine.

You now need to learn to keep the lower stomach muscles engaged while you breathe in and out, otherwise you will lose your core stability while attempting an exercise like the Single Leg Stretch (page 170). To do this you need to be able to breathe laterally.

▷ Breathe in to prepare. Lengthen up through the top of your head.
▷ Breathe out and draw the lower abdominals back towards the spine, hollowing out your lower stomach.
▷ Breathe in to your sides allowing your ribcage to expand fully, keeping the stomach hollowed out and firm.
▷ Continue to breathe in and out, maintaining the strong centre.

You may also like to try finding the core muscles on the pause between the out-breath and the in-breath:

▷ Breathe in to prepare.
▷ Breathe out completely.
▷ Then, engage the lower abdominals.
▷ Breathe in, keeping the abdominals hollowed.

This is not the way that Pilates taught 'navel to spine' but we have found it useful in teaching isolation of the deep abdominals.

You will notice that we have chosen to use the word 'hollow' to describe the action. It is very important that you do not grip your abdominals tightly, for this will only create unnecessary tension and you will probably engage the wrong muscles to boot. Think of:

▷ Hollowing
▷ Scooping
▷ Drawing back . . . the abdominals towards the spine

Have you found the right muscles yet? Another way to find them is on all fours (see page 36):

▷ Kneel on all fours, your hands beneath your shoulders and shoulder-width apart.
▷ Your knees are beneath your hips. Have the top of your head lengthening away from your tailbone. Your pelvis is in neutral.
▷ Breathe in to prepare.
▷ Breathe out, and draw the lower abdominals up towards the spine. Your back should not move.

▷ Breathe in and release.

▷ Practice eight times and then try keeping the abdominals hollowed for both the out- and the in-breath.

Still having trouble finding them?

▷ Lie on your front. Rest your head on your folded hands, opening the shoulders out and relaxing the upper back. You may need a small, flat cushion under your abdomen if your low back is uncomfortable. Your legs are shoulder-width apart and turned out, your feet long.

▷ Breathe in to prepare, breathe out and lift the lower abdominals off the floor. Imagine there is a precious egg under them that must not be crushed.

▷ Breathe in and release.

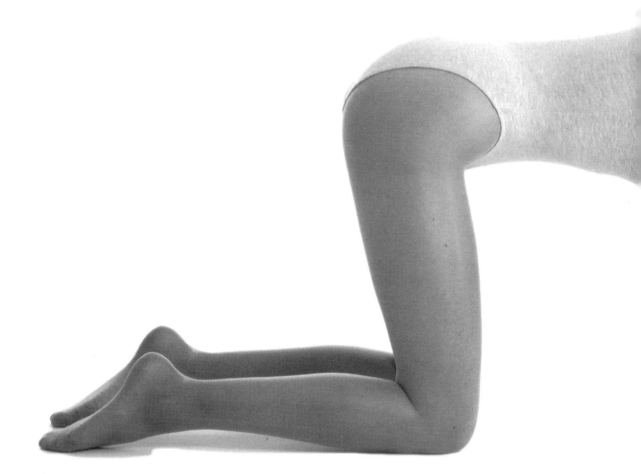

All fours

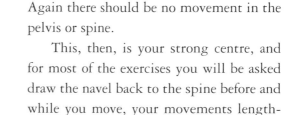

Precious egg

Again there should be no movement in the pelvis or spine.

This, then, is your strong centre, and for most of the exercises you will be asked draw the navel back to the spine before and while you move, your movements lengthening away from a strong centre.

When you have mastered this technique, you should try to add lifting from the pelvic floor at the same time (see page 76).

Please note that for ease of language we refer to the 'navel' being drawn back to the spine, which is how Joseph Pilates described it. Technically, we should always say 'lower abdominals' as the action is low in the abdomen.

Good Upper Body Use

We have already discussed the muscle imbalances that are caused by habitual poor posture, reflecting again on the use of the upper body. We are aiming to open the chest, which is frequently tight, relax the upper shoulder and neck muscles and encourage the use of the mid-back muscles around the lower part of the shoulder blades.

While you are exercising, it is very easy to forget what is happening in this area. Often, and without realizing it, your neck is doing the work that your abdominals should be doing. Your shoulders become tense and end up around your ears.

These simple rules will help you to overcome this and can be applied to many of the exercises in this book as well as those of other fitness programmes.

▷ Keep your shoulder blades down into your back
▷ Your neck released
▷ Your breastbone soft
▷ Your elbows open

Good Upper Body Use

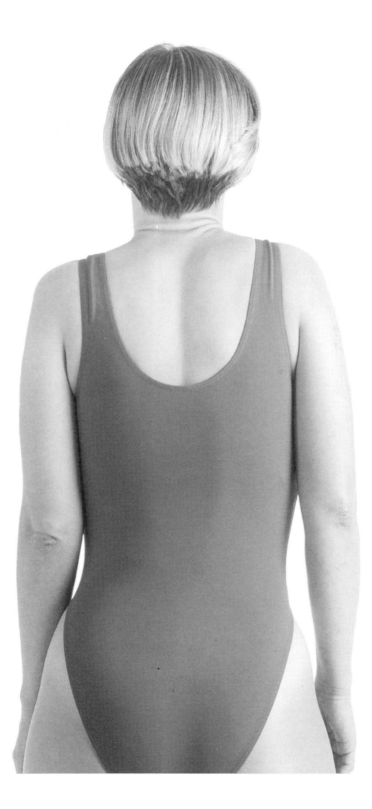

Bad Upper Body Use

Explorations and

Exercises

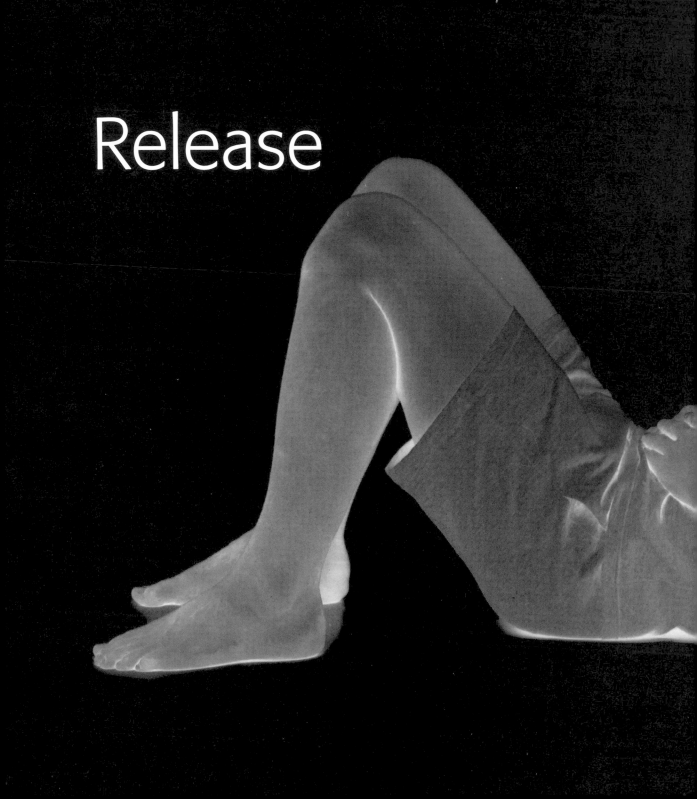

Release

The word '**stress**' comes from the Latin *stressere*, to bind tightly. It is stress that has many of us tied up securely in knots, so this chapter is all about **untying those knots**.

Release

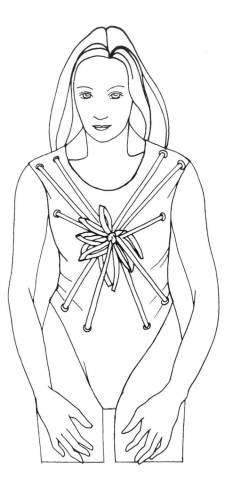

'fight or flight' response to danger: 'Do I stay and fight the hairy mammoth or do I run away? Either way, I'm going to need all my senses sharpened, all my strength to tackle the enemy.'

So, the adrenaline pumps, the pulse quickens, blood pressure rises. Meanwhile, all other 'non urgent' bodily functions shut down so that you can concentrate on the danger, which is why, when you are scared, you feel nauseous (or worse), for the body does not want to waste energy digesting food, in view of the more pressing matters it has to cope with.

This is a great system which has helped our survival but, as we have seen, it can work against us. If the stress is sustained and not turned off, these basic bodily functions do not function efficiently – they remain in 'shut down' mode. In particular, our auto repair system – our immune system – is interrupted.

As we have already noted, in the absence of the mammoth, we have substituted other stresses such as work problems, marital problems and meeting publishers' deadlines – the daily hassles we all face. Some of us handle these external pressures

Let's consider our forebears once again. We have already discussed how their daily survival required that they have a sophisticated

very well but many react inappropriately for it is hard to solve such stresses because they are often very complex and we cannot fight them head on, scare them away or turn them off. The results are very physical and range from a breakdown of the immune system, stomach ulcers, allergic reactions, kidney disease, irritable bowel, high blood pressure and tension headaches to heart conditions and cancer.

But how do we break the cycle?

The first step is learning how to let go, how to relax and release. If you can learn to release the tension in muscles, the brain will pick up the message that all is well, the danger (and therefore the stress) is passed and the body can revert to normal – and this includes the immune system.

With tension released, we can then start to build on sound movement patterns. In any fitness programme it is vital to relax and lengthen any short or tight muscles before attempting to strengthen the weak ones. Why?

We have already mentioned how most of us suffer from muscle imbalances (page 24). If we tried to strengthen any of the weaker muscles before we had allowed the short tight muscles to lengthen, then the latter would only prevent any good movement pattern. We know that muscles work in groups to produce movement, some contracting and working, others releasing and

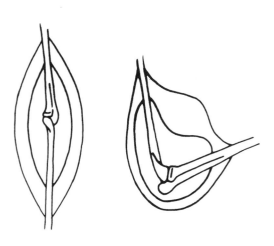

Muscles work in pairs to move bones

lengthening to allow for that contraction to take place.

All the members of that group need to be able to fulfil their role if the movement sequence is to be efficient. If one muscle is too tight, its opposing partner or partners will not be able to function correctly. Therefore, we cannot even begin to introduce sound body use until these short, overactive muscles have been released and lengthened.

The following explorations and exercises have been designed to help you to release tension in every part of your body, opening the joints, keeping them open, releasing to expand, lengthen, widen. This is 'letting go', letting the body and mind come to a state of ease.

Relaxation Position

This position is used extensively in the Alexander Technique, where it is called the Semi Supine Position or Constructive Rest. It enables you to release tension and tight muscles in a gravity-reduced setting. This means that it is easier for you to explore where you might be holding unnecessary tension as you do not have to worry about losing control and so, for example, falling over.

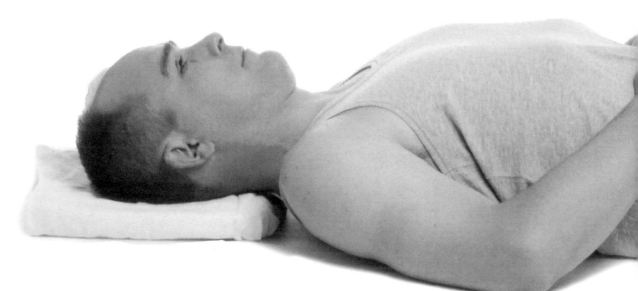

Semi Supine or Relaxation Position

While you are resting in this position your spine is gradually lengthening, mainly as a result of releasing the muscles in your back and, more specifically, around your spinal column. The tiny building blocks of your spine, called vertebrae, are cushioned by intervertebral discs which act very much like shock absorbers. The name 'disc' is rather misleading as it suggests solid matter, whilst discs are, in reality, fluid-filled, spongy pouches looking very much like jelly. As a result of gravitational pull, bad

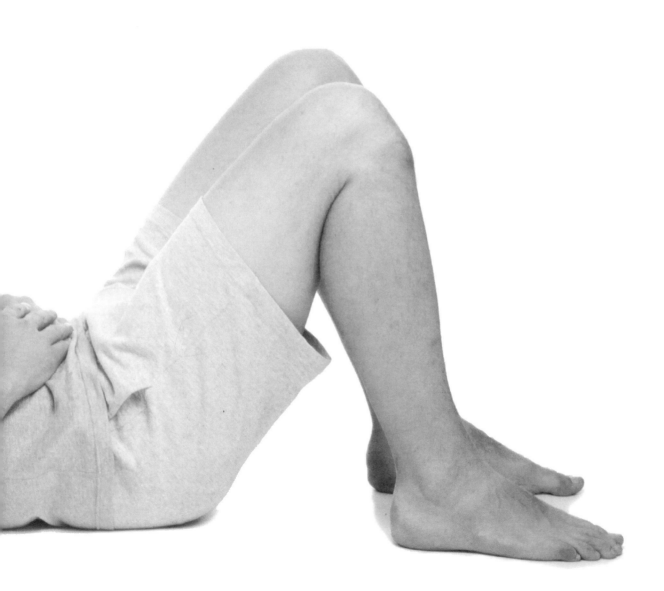

posture and alignment or old age these discs get squashed and they decrease in size, resulting in a shortened spinal column. Therefore, we are taller in youth and 'shrink' in old age.

While relaxing in this position for approximately twenty minutes, gravity will help your muscles to relax and, as a result, your spine can fully lengthen as the discs are filling with fluid.

Please note that it is inadvisable to remain in this position for any length of time after your second term of pregnancy.

Preparation

You will need:
A small firm pillow or a paperback book.
A slightly cushioned or padded surface to lie on (most beds are too soft).

▷ Lie on your side in a foetal position, knees into your chest, your head on the pillow or book.
▷ During your next out-breath, roll gently on to your back while keeping your knees into your chest.
▷ Place your feet in line with your hips, one at a time, on the floor.
▷ Keep your toes parallel and your heels in line with the centre of your buttocks.
▷ Keep your toes in the same line – you might initially need someone to check this for you.

▷ Let your shoulders widen and your elbows open by placing your hands on your abdomen. You are now ready to start the exercise.

Action

A big part of this exercise is about active non-doing – it is like going inside your body and exploring the space within. Doing less is doing more during this exercise.

▷ Allow your feet to melt into the floor. Let them spread and distribute the weight evenly throughout the whole foot.
▷ Allow the ankle to soften and pay particular attention to releasing the front of your ankle.
▷ Allow the weight of your legs to transfer into your hip socket and your feet. Use a minimal amount of muscular tension to keep your legs in this position. Release, in particular, the front of your thighs and where the thighbone connects on to your pelvis.
▷ Check how relaxed your hip flexors are by gently letting the legs go from side to side.
▷ Allow your back to sink into the floor and lengthen.
▷ Allow your buttocks to spread and support your pelvis.
▷ Let your shoulders melt towards the ground, imagining your collar bones spreading out towards the shoulder

joint like the wings of a bird. Imagine your breast bone softening and gently sinking towards the spine.

▷ Be aware of the rise and fall of your abdomen. Notice how every in-breath gently widens your back and how the out-breath contracts the whole rib cage.

▷ Allow yourself to be supported by the floor.

▷ Release the back of your head into the pillow-book, keeping your face parallel to the ceiling. Imagine that there is lots of air under your chin. Avoid making double chins or tilting your head back and shortening your neck.

▷ Release your tongue, letting it fully spread in your mouth, releasing it at the back where it attaches to your throat.

▷ Release your face, softening the muscles, allowing the eyes to float in their sockets and the brain to rest in the skull.

From Lying to Standing

Letting your knees roll over to one side, is the most elegant and easiest way to transfer from a lying position to standing. You should use this technique all the time, especially when getting out of bed. Keeping your head and neck relaxed:

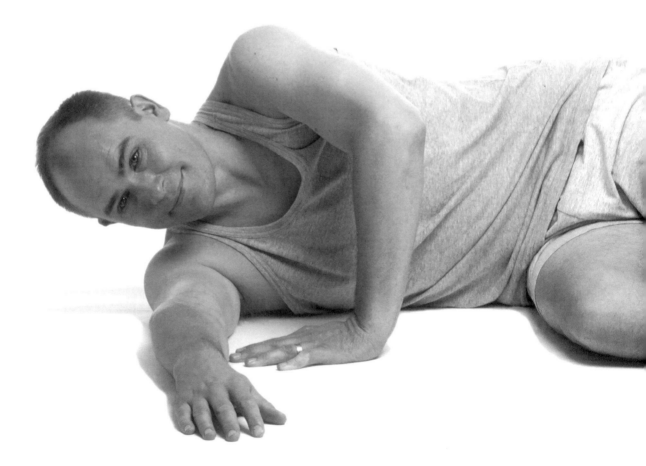

▷ Let your knees gently roll the whole of your body to one side.

▷ You are now in the foetal position, resting fully on your side.

▷ Use your arms and hands to come to a sitting position, gently parting your legs sideways in a scissors-like position.

▷ Bring up one knee at a time, supporting your torso with your hands on the floor, coming up in a spiral-like movement.

Tense and Release

This exploration is the first step towards learning to let go. It is one of the ways to release areas that are very tight. Muscles can only contract and release. Therefore, it is sometimes useful to tighten a muscle even more, mentally register the tightness and then let go.

While you are learning this routine, it may be worth asking a friend to read the actions to you. Be patient for, although this exploration may easily take up to thirty minutes initially, after practice and memorizing the basic sequence, you will find that the same result can be achieved in five to ten minutes. You will find it much easier to pinpoint tight zones and, indeed, to 'connect'.

Preparation

You can either adopt the semi-supine position or you might prefer to lie on your back with a rolled-up duvet under your knees. This might help you, initially, to be able to concentrate better.

Action

▷ Start by becoming aware of your feet, especially the soles and the toes.

▷ Squeeze the whole of your foot tightly, during your next in-breath. When you exhale let go of all the muscles in the foot.

▷ Repeat three times. Every time you let go, imagine how all the tension flows away. Send your awareness into your calves. Notice how the muscles rest on the floor, supporting your leg.

▷ On your next in-breath squeeze the muscles very tightly to the bone and then let go again during your out-breath.

▷ Repeat this action three times, noticing how the muscles are softening more and more after every squeeze. Imagine how the tendons at the back of your knee are softening, enabling the knee to 'open'.

▷ Become aware of your thigh muscles, including the hamstrings at the back of your thighs. Tighten the muscles, squeeze as hard as you can – muscle to bone. Release again on your next out-breath.

▷ Repeat three times.

▷ Notice how the whole leg gently rolls out from your hip joint. Send your thoughts into your buttocks. Notice how they spread on the floor supporting your pelvis – the buttock muscles are the largest muscles in the body. Squeeze and release, repeating three times.

▷ Imagine your pelvis being a bony bowl, containing vital organs. Let your next out-breath soften the bones and, as a result, the bowl is widening, providing more space for everything contained inside.

▷ Send your awareness into your spine, from the tailbone all the way up into your skull. Let the muscles in your back give off all the unwanted tensions into the floor. As a result, the whole of your back is lengthening and, with every breath you take, widening.

▷ Let your attention focus on your arms. From the shoulder joint into the upper arm, into the elbow, reaching the forearm, travelling into the hand, all the way into the tips of your fingers. Repeat the squeezing and releasing as above.

▷ From the arms, let your mind travel into your neck and head. The next out-breath melts the tightness, smoothes the forehead and especially releases the jaw muscles.

Standing Release

Aim

To find postural alignment with the added difficulty of the dynamic pull towards gravity.

Preparation

▷ Stand comfortably with your feet hip-width apart, your feet parallel.

▷ Gently release your knees, unlocking them.

▷ Let your arms hang comfortably by your side.

▷ Keep breathing at your natural rate and look straight ahead, not tucking the chin under or throwing the head back, thereby contracting your neck.

Relax your weight through the bones of the skeleton, working with gravity.

Release your head upwards, towards the ceiling, lengthening the spine.

Imagine your head as effortlessly balancing on top of your spine.

Let your tailbone gently drop towards the floor as if you had a weight attached to it, but still maintaining the natural neutral spine/pelvis position (see page 30).

Note the level of tension in your thighs. Release any that is not necessary to keep you in this upright position. To check, you can gently move your knees from side to side. You should notice constant slight movements throughout your body, as it adjusts to finding its natural balance.

Spread your feet on the floor, distributing the weight evenly.

The Sunbathing Spider

Aim

To bring you in touch with your back and to release tension in the musculature around your spine and ribcage.

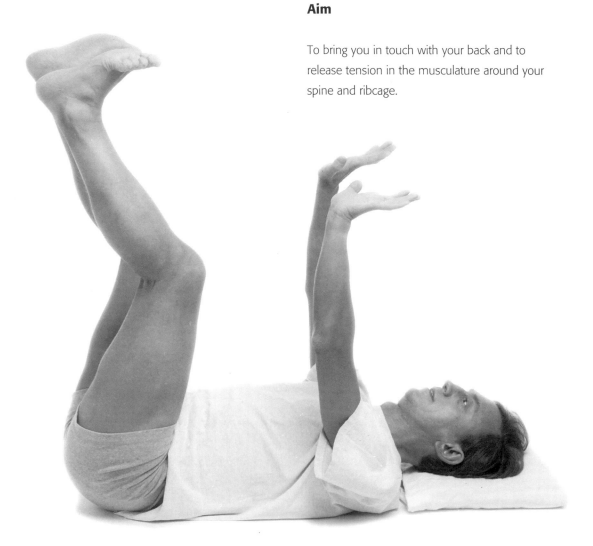

Sunbathing Spider

Preparation

Lie on your back on a mat or a slightly padded surface to protect your spine and vertebrae.

Action

▷ Stretch your arms to the ceiling at a right angle.

▷ Bend your knees on to your chest one at a time and then straighten them slowly towards the ceiling, keeping them hip-width apart. Make sure that your tailbone stays firmly on the ground!

▷ Flex your feet, as if you where showing the soles of your feet to the ceiling.

▷ Keep breathing at your own pace.

▷ Feel yourself 'anchored' to the floor, the shoulder blades widening, the low back releasing.

To Finish

▷ Let your arms cross over your chest, as if you were hugging yourself.

▷ Let your legs hang, let your ankles cross over and your heels come close to your backside.

▷ Be aware of the contact of your back with the floor – has it changed? Be aware of your breath.

▷ Take care to lower your legs slowly to the floor, one at a time, with a strong centre.

Note

If holding your legs in this position is too strenuous for your stomach muscles, try it with your feet up a wall, or with a friend holding your ankles for you.

Roll Downs

Aim

To release tension in the spine, the shoulders and the upper body. To mobilize the spine, creating flexibility and strength. To teach correct use of abdominals when bending.

Preparation

▷ Stand with your feet hip-width apart and in parallel, your weight evenly balanced on both feet.

▷ Check that you are not rolling your feet in or out.

▷ Soft knees.

▷ Find your neutral pelvis position but keep the tailbone lengthening down.

▷ Draw your navel back to the spine.

▷ Lengthen up through the top of your head

▷ Shoulders widening.

▷ Arms relaxing.

Action

▷ Breathe in to prepare and lengthen up through the spine, release the head and neck.

▷ Breathe out, and draw the lower abdominals back towards the spine.

▷ Drop your chin on to your chest and allow the weight of your head to make you slowly roll forward, head released, arms hanging, centre strong, knees soft (see note).

▷ Breathe in as you hang, really letting your head and arms hang.

▷ Breathe out, navel firmly back to spine as you drop down your tailbone, directing your pubic bone forward. Rotate your pelvis as you slowly come up to standing tall, rolling through the spine bone by bone.

▷ Repeat six times.

You may like to take an extra breath during the exercise. This is fine but please try to breathe out as you move the spine .

Note

Take care if you have back problems – keep your knees very bent or try sitting in a chair. You may also prefer to include this exercise towards the end of a session when you are well warmed-up and the spine is freer.

If you have a disc-related problem, please consult your medical practitioner first.

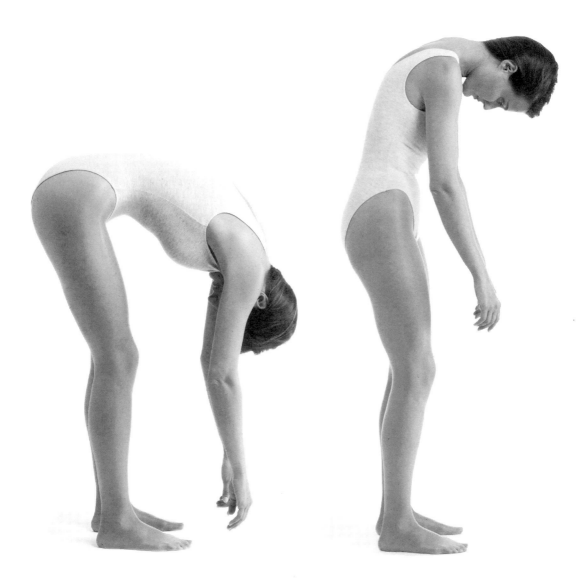

Fully down   *Halfway up*

Zigzags

Aim

To 'open' the hips, the knees and the ankle joints. To learn to turn the legs in and out.

Preparation

You will need a small flat pillow.

▷ Lie on the floor about half a metre away from a clear wall space. Your hips should be square to the wall, your head resting on the pillow.

▷ Place the feet together on the wall so that your knees form a right angle. Check that your pelvis is in a neutral position.

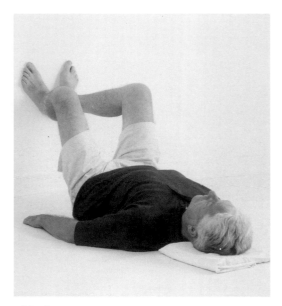

Slide the toes apart

Action

▷ Slide your toes apart as far as they go, keeping the heels together.

▷ Now, keeping the balls of the feet still, slide the heels apart as far as they go.

▷ Continue zigzagging the feet in this

way, making certain that they stay flat on the wall. You should be transferring the weight of the feet alternately through the heels and then through the balls of the feet.

▷ Zigzag until the feet refuse to turn any more. The legs are as wide as you can comfortably open them, without changing your pelvic alignment. Then zigzag back together again.

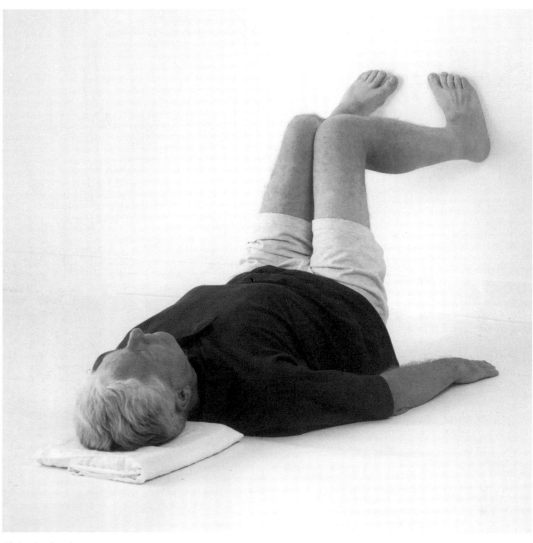

Slide the heels apart

Awareness Points

▷ Check to see that the level of your feet has not dropped and that both feet are at the same height.

▷ Please try not to lift the feet off the wall. You are pivoting alternately on the balls and heels but letting the feet slide.

▷ Keep neutral!

Knee Bends

Aim

To release tension around the hip joint. To learn correct muscle use in the pelvic area.

Preparation

You will need a scarf or belt – otherwise, wear baggy tracksuit leggings that you can hold on to.

▷ Lie on your back in the Relaxation Position.

▷ Tie the scarf loosely around one thigh so that you can easily hold it while moving the leg.

▷ Check that your pelvis is in neutral.

▷ Take hold of one leg.

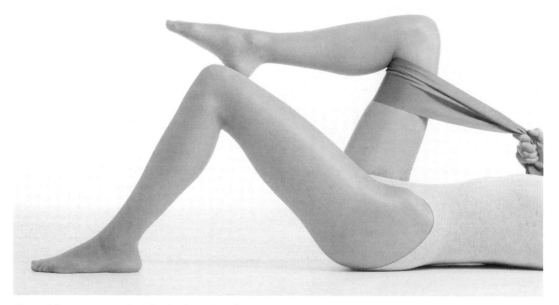

The pelvis stays neutral while the knee bends

Action

▷ Breathe in to prepare.

▷ Breathe out, hollow the lower abdominals and, with the help of your hand, fold one knee up. Think of dropping the thigh bone down into the hip socket. Try to keep the length in the front of your pelvis. The lower back may drop a little into the floor but you should ensure that the tailbone stays lengthening away down on the floor. The pelvis should stay neutral.

▷ Breathe in.

▷ Breathe out, hollow, and slowly unfold the knee back on to the floor.

▷ Repeat eight times with each leg.

▷ When you can fold the knee comfortably, you may bend the knee without the guidance of your hand. Try to remember the feeling of this movement for when you are doing other exercises, such as the Single Leg Stretch on page 170.

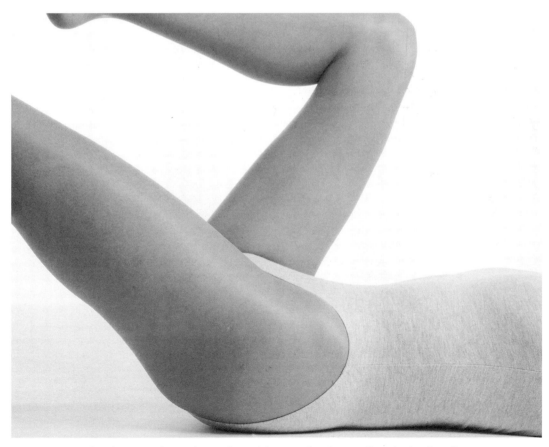

Incorrect Knee Bend. Remember to leave the pelvis neutral – do not allow the back to flatten.

Awareness

'The **body** has a great ability to **readjust** and **heal itself** and usually reacts correctly and therapeutically if given the chance and encouragement. **Increased sensory awareness** and **sensitivity** make it possible to obtain more and better information as to the states of **body and mind**; good judgement will suggest what ought to be done; and **willpower** will ensure that it is done.'

Jencks

Awareness

In the last chapter, we looked at the first stage in re-educating the body – letting go. The next stage involves learning how to react appropriately to external stimuli, to be aware of how your body is responding and to learn how to decide and choose anew instead of acting out of habit.

The starting point for learning how to respond is, perhaps surprisingly, not to respond – at least for a moment. 'Active non-doing' sounds like a contradiction in terms, yet it does require a lot of thought to stop the body and mind reacting to a given stimuli. Take an example – the ringing tone of a telephone can trigger certain responses in people, which are totally inappropriate and unnecessary. Just observe the way that you react next time the telephone rings. You will be amazed at how tense your body can go, your head will drop back and your neck muscles tighten (this was originally to protect the brain). All this, and it was only a double glazing salesman!

So, most of us react to specific situations in a way that might potentially harm us, sometimes physically and sometimes mentally. 'Active non-doing' is very much like stopping to let something new, a new way of being, moving and even feeling and thinking, take place.

▷ It is like making space for change.
▷ It is like a pause we have to create to let the flow of life change direction.

This is very difficult and sometimes very painful, not only on a physical level. Change is frightening, for sometimes we only have the way we react and live our life to hold on to.

Taking a moment to pause before we react is no good if we then go on to move in the same way with the same bad habits. We therefore have to learn new, better habits, better ways of moving that do not abuse the body. The way we use our bodies, minds – and, to a certain degree, we can also include emotions – is very much determined by habit. This feels comfortable, it feels like home, like being you. Quite often we react almost automatically, as if we were not thinking. This does not usually cause a problem and it only becomes apparent when we are physically in pain or have emotional problems.

These habits can be so strong that it is very difficult to imagine life without them, and that is fine providing that you are happy in the way you are. Most people will instinctively say 'yes' if asked whether they are happy with themselves but, interestingly, it seems to be the body in the first instance that gives signs of 'dis-ease' or, in a lesser degree, pain and discomfort. W. Reich, a psychoanalyst, was the first in his field to recognize the immediate effect of the mind and emotions on the body and vice versa. Muscles store memories and past experiences, which the mind sometimes has to push aside or 'choose' to forget. Reich believed that a person consists of mind, body, spirit and emotions. However, the four elements are interlocked, continually reacting to each other and influencing each other. Emotions are part of us and we can feel them physically in our bodies and, in the same way, the state of our body can change the way that we feel.

Unreliable or faulty sensory awareness

When muscles become shortened, the brain will receive information about this altered state via the sensory neurones, which are situated in the joints, muscles and tendons. They 'measure' stretch or contraction and send this information via the sensory nerve cells to the brain. If a muscle is continually shortened there is no new information for the brain to receive and register. As a result, the sensory mechanism goes to sleep because it has nothing to do!

This can create an interesting phenomenon, for the process of muscles returning to their optimum length can be experienced as very unpleasant. When the body returns to a more balanced state the sensory feedback to the brain 'wakes up' once more, transmitting the changes that occur. This results in floods of new sensations which may either feel delightful or, alternatively, very strange and unfamiliar.

Change should happen gradually, to allow muscles to stretch and strengthen and joints to move more freely. One's sensory awareness becomes more reliable as it gradually changes and redevelops.

This next set of explorations and exercises should put you more in touch with your body. They will help develop your sensory awareness, your body's own 'biofeedback' system, known as your kinaesthetic sense. By improving your sensory awareness, you will be able to read more accurately the messages of the body, to detect 'stressors' before they become harmful. You can learn how to identify, sense and feel anew and then respond appropriately.

Landmarks of Alignment

Aim

To become more familiar with the bony landmarks of the body. To be able to have a tactile experience of alignment.

Action

▷ Stand in a balanced position.

▷ Using your fingers, touch the centre of each ear, while letting the elbows extend horizontally. Imagine the fingers meeting in the centre of your skull – this is the place where the skull balances on top of your spine. You can get a better feel for this if you gently nod your head.

▷ Let your hands move downwards to the sides of your ribcage, thumbs behind, fingers in front. Be aware of the oval-like shape of your ribs and how each breath expands and contracts that three-dimensional cage.

▷ Place your hands on the sides of your pelvis and, from there, gently glide them down the outside of your legs. At the top of your leg you will come across a bony projection – this is part of your thighbone and is larger in women than in men.

▷ Let your hands stroke downwards along the side of your leg until you are touching the sides of your knees.

▷ Continue towards your feet, touching the bumps on the outside of each ankle. Touch the floor.

▷ Bring your fingers around and touch the second toe on both feet. Draw imaginary lines from your second toe through the centre of each ankle, heel, knee, the centre of each hip socket (which is deeply embedded in your pelvis).

▷ Repeat this several times to trace the parallel alignment of feet, ankles, knees and pelvis.

▷ You finish this exercise by stroking from the pelvis up the side of the ribs, the side of your head and up further into the air.

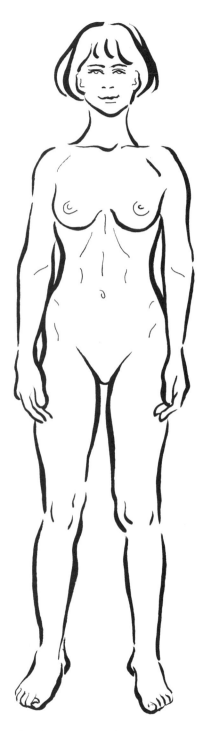
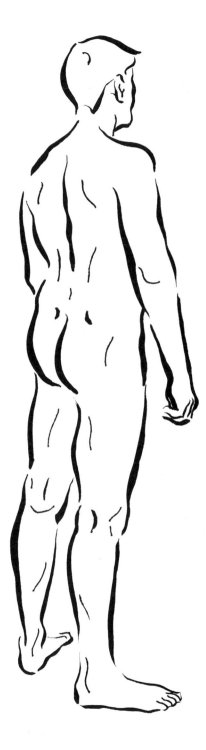

The bony landmarks of your body

Floating Shoulders

This exercise, along with the Opening Doors, Shoulder Presses and the Diamond Press, is a key exercise in developing the strength of the mid-back muscles which stabilize the scapulae, enabling the neck to be free.

Aim

To be aware of using the appropriate muscles of the shoulder girdle, while keeping other muscles 'quiet', that is, actively not engaging these other muscles. We are aiming to minimize the workload of the upper trapezius which tends to overwork and can thus cause great tension in the neck and shoulders.

Preparation

You may need a mirror to help you check that you are doing the exercise correctly.

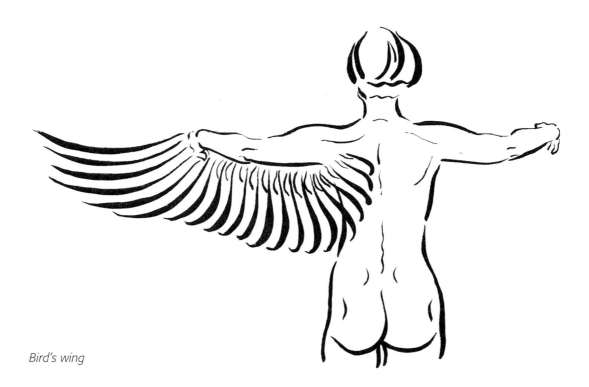

Bird's wing

▷ Stand easily (see page 54), or you may sit on a chair.

▷ Place your right hand on your left shoulder, your left arm hanging by your side, the palm angled, facing forward.

Action

▷ Breathe in to prepare and lengthen up through the spine, letting the neck be free.

▷ Breathe out, navel to spine, and slowly begin to raise the arm reaching wide out of the shoulderblades like a bird's wing. Think of the hand as leading the arm, the arm following the hand as it

floats upwards. You will need to rotate the arm so that the palm opens to the ceiling as the arm reaches shoulder level. Try to keep the shoulder under your hand as still as possible and the shoulderblades connecting and dropping down into your back as long as possible.

▷ Breathe in as you lower the arm to your side.

▷ Repeat on the other side.

▷ As soon as you feel that you have mastered keeping the shoulders down while raising the arm and using the shoulderblades correctly, you can try raising both arms together. Check in the mirror that you are doing the exercise correctly.

Opening Doors

Aim

To become aware of the shoulderblades and their positioning. To work the muscles between and below the shoulderblades, keeping the upper shoulder muscles relaxed.

Preparation

▷ Stand easily or sit on the edge of a chair.

▷ Hold your arms out to the side in line with your shoulders. Bend your arms

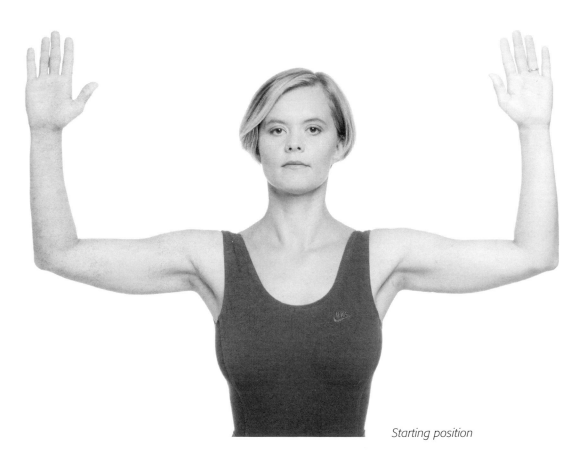

Starting position

at the elbows at a right angle, your palms face forwards.

Action

▷ Breathe in to prepare and lengthen up through the spine. Breathe out, navel to spine, and move the arms forward in front of you until they meet, fingers to elbows touching. Your elbows should be in a line with the centre of your chest. Notice what has happened to your shoulderblades – they will have opened out. Your mid back is also widening.

▷ Breathe in as you bring your arms back to the starting position, opening the chest. Again, notice the movement of your shoulderblades – they will have closed back together again.
Repeat five times.

Awareness Points

▷ Be aware of any tension in your neck, gently release it.
▷ Remember to keep the shoulderblades down into your back.

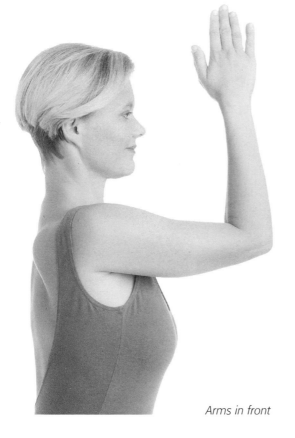

Arms in front

Shoulder Presses

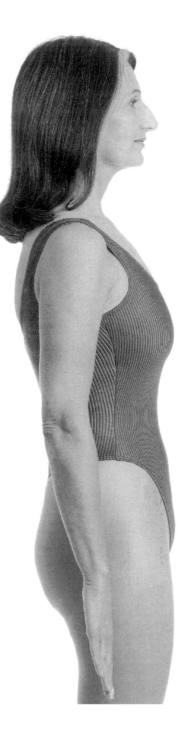

Aim

To increase awareness of the shoulderblades and the muscles around them. To work the muscles which stabilize the shoulderblades.

Preparation

You may either stand for this exercise or you may sit on a straight-backed chair, your feet firmly planted on the floor, hip-width apart and the knees at right angles. Your arms arc by your sides, palms facing backwards.

Starting position

Action

▷ Breathe in and lengthen up through the spine, shoulders relaxed.

▷ Breathe out, draw navel to spine, and push the palms backwards as far as is comfortable. Keep your neck soft. Be aware of the muscles between the shoulder blades working.

▷ Breathe in and release.

▷ Repeat five times.

Awareness Points

▷ Keep those shoulderblades down and into your back.

▷ Do not fully straighten your elbows, keep them soft.

▷ Release your neck throughout the exercise.

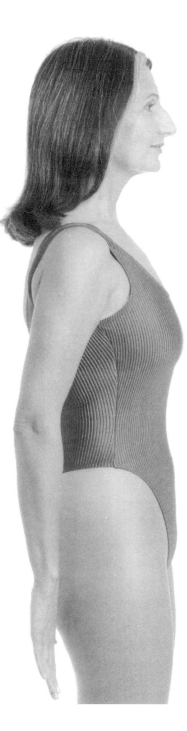

Arms back

The Pelvic Floor

The muscles of the pelvic floor are an often neglected area when exercising and yet the muscular sling that they form supports and holds the pelvic organs, bladder, rectum and womb in place. Quite a task!

There are many reasons why these muscles weaken. For women, however, the main cause of weakness is pregnancy and childbirth. Gentlemen, you cannot remain complacent, however, because these muscles are equally important for you as, in particular, they can help with prostate problems. By strengthening these muscles, men and women can expect the following benefits:

▷ Fewer problems with incontinence and prolapse.
▷ Better sexual relations.
▷ Better 'core stability'. These muscles act with the abdominal muscles to maintain intra-abdominal pressure during exertion, in that they also have a role to play in supporting the back.
▷ Fewer prostate problems for men and help in treatment.

The most obvious time for extra pelvic floor exercises – and usually the only time most women are ever given them to do – is after childbirth. And yet we should all be doing these exercises regularly..

There is just one cautionary note. As with all the other muscles, we are looking for a perfect balance of strength, flexibility and control. You need to be able to let go as well as tighten, something which is especially true during pregnancy. The last thing you want are pelvic floor muscles which are so tight that they will not release during the birth itself. The 'Flower' exercise is a wonderful way of teaching you how to open this area in preparation for the final stages of labour.

One other point: you may have been told that stopping the stream of urine in mid-flow is a way of testing the strength of these muscles. It is very important that you do not use this as an exercise, for it is to be regarded as a test only and should not be practised regularly because urinary infections may result. You may, of course, use it as a way of finding the right muscles, which is what the first exercises below are all about.

Figure of Eight

Before you can begin to work the pelvic floor, we have to find the right muscles.

Aim

To isolate and activate the muscles of the pelvic floor openings, while keeping the rest of the body relaxed.

Preparation

Sit squarely on a chair, your feet hip-width apart and flat on the floor (use a cushion under them if necessary). Check that your pelvis is in neutral, your spine long and your shoulders relaxed.

Action

▷ Take your awareness down to your pelvic floor.
▷ Breathe out and try to close the urethra (front passage from which you pass urine).
▷ Breathe in and check that your shoulders are still relaxed.
▷ Breathe out and, still lifting from the front, try to close the muscles around the anus (back passage) keeping your buttocks relaxed!
▷ Breathe in, and double check that your shoulders and jaw are soft.
▷ Breathe out, and add lifting from the vagina (gentlemen, please improvise).
▷ Breathe in and hold all three.
▷ As you breathe out, gently release the muscles.
▷ Practice three times.

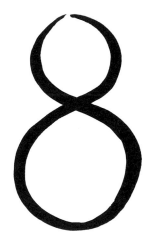

The Figure of Eight representing your pelvic floor

We never said it was easy! If you are still struggling to find the pelvic muscles, you could try sitting on your hand and trying to detect a change in pressure.

The Pelvic Elevator

In this exercise you will be lifting the whole of the pelvic floor together.

Preparation

Sit as above – you can, in fact, do these exercises in any position. Imagine that the whole of the pelvic floor area – front, back and middle – is a lift in a building.

Action

▷ Breathe in to prepare.
▷ Breathe out, and lift the pelvic floor just a little to bring it up to the first floor of your building.
▷ Breathe in.
▷ Breathe out, and lift the pelvic floor to the second floor of the building.
▷ Breathe in.
▷ Breathe out, and bring the lift to the third floor.
▷ Breathe in.
▷ If you have a penthouse suite you may go higher! Otherwise, bring the lift back down, floor by floor, until you reach the ground floor again when you can completely release. Just check that your shoulders do not end up around your ears with this one. Try not to clench the buttocks.
▷ Practice three times.

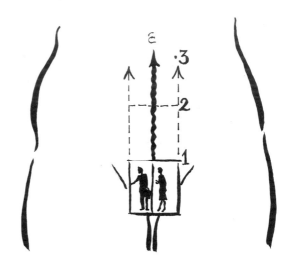

The Pelvic Elevator

The Flower

Aim

To work the muscles of the pelvic floor and, equally importantly, to learn how to release them.

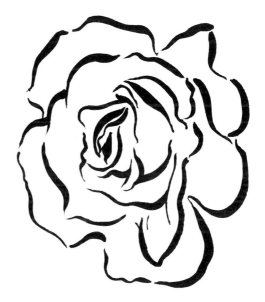

Action

▷ Gradually draw the pelvic floor up and in, just like a flower closing at the end of the day.

▷ Now, gradually release the muscles, letting them open like a flower opening in the morning sun.

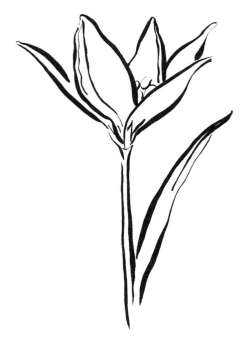

The Emergency Stop

Ever been caught short if you cough or sneeze? This is one to practice, if you have.

Action

▷ Simply lift the whole of the pelvic floor, tightening it all quickly as if in an emergency.

▷ Hold for about five seconds, then release.

▷ Practice five times.

The Squeezes: The Big Squeeze

Aim

To work the muscles of the lower abdomen, pelvic floor, the buttocks and the inner thighs, keeping the upper body relaxed.

Preparation

▷ Lie on your front.
▷ Place, or get a close friend to, a small cushion between the tops of your thighs.

▷ Rest your forehead on your folded hands, open and relax the shoulders.
▷ Have your toes together and your heels apart.

Action

▷ Breathe in to prepare.
▷ Breathe out, draw the lower abdominals up to the spine as if there is a fragile egg under the stomach and you do not wish to crush it.

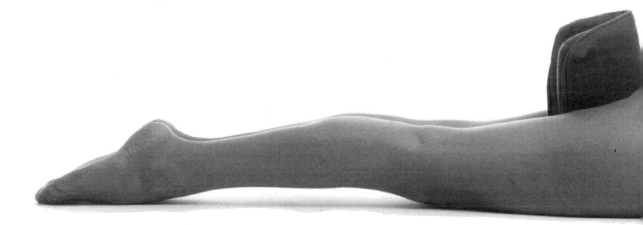

- ▷ Breathe in and release.
- ▷ Breathe out and lift the stomach again, but now add the lifting from the pelvic floor as well.
- ▷ Breathe in and release.
- ▷ Breathe out, lift the stomach, the pelvic floor and now add tightening the buttocks, squeezing the inner thighs and the cushion and bringing the heels together! Hold for a count of five. *Keep breathing normally and continually check that you are only working from the waist down.*
- ▷ Then release.
- ▷ Repeat the Big Squeeze five times.

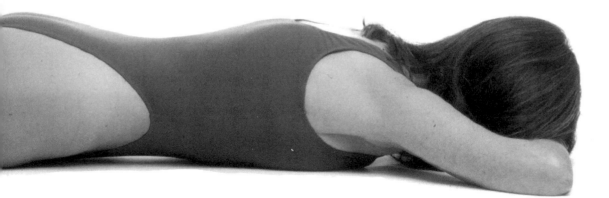

The Pillow Squeeze

Preparation

You will need a large pillow.

▷ Lie on your back, your knees bent, feet together and flat on the floor, arms by your side.
▷ Open the knees and place the folded pillow between them.
▷ Double check that your pelvis is in neutral.

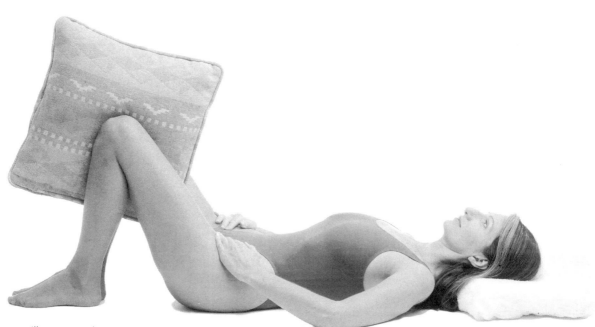

Pillow squeezing

Action

▷ Breathe in deeply to prepare.

▷ Breathe out, hollowing out the lower abdominals. Do not tuck the pelvis or engage the muscles around the hips.

▷ Now lift the pelvic floor and squeeze the knees and inner thighs together.

▷ Breathing normally now, hold the squeeze for the count of a minimum of six and a maximum of ten before releasing.

▷ Repeat five times.

Awareness Points

▷ Don't let your neck join in the action – think of softening the breastbone and neck as you squeeze.

▷ Nine out of ten people tilt their pelvis to North on this exercise so, concentrate on keeping your tailbone down and lengthening away, keeping the length between the navel and the pubic bone. You can try placing your hand under your waist to check that you are not pushing into the spine.

▷ Try placing your hands where your leg joins the front of your pelvis, that is, at your hip joint. You are trying to keep this area relaxed.

▷ If you suffer from sciatica, try squeezing the pillow just with the tips of your knees. It helps to release the sciatic nerve in your back.

Adductor Openings

The adductor muscles are very important postural muscles which need to be kept strong but long.

Aim

To stretch the adductor muscles which run along the inside of your thighs down to your knees.

Preparation

Adopt the Relaxation Position.

Action

▷ Bring both knees up on to your chest, one at a time. Place one hand under each thigh and then allow the legs to slowly open.

▷ Breathe normally as you allow gravity to stretch out the muscles .

▷ Hold this position for a couple of minutes. Then slowly close the legs and return the feet to the floor one at a time with the navel to spine.

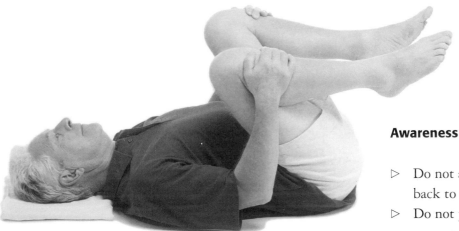

Awareness Points

▷ Do not allow your back to over-arch.

▷ Do not put too much pressure on the knees.

Quadriceps Lengthening

Aim

To lengthen gently the quadriceps at the front of the thigh.

Please avoid this exercise if you have knee problems.

Preparation

Lie on your front, your forehead resting on your folded hands. Check that your shoulders are completely relaxed.

Action

▷ Breathe in to prepare.

▷ Breathe out, navel to spine.

▷ Alternately kick your right leg and left leg into your bottom, flexing the foot as you do so.

▷ Breathe normally, keeping your abdominals hollowed throughout.

▷ Repeat ten times on each leg.

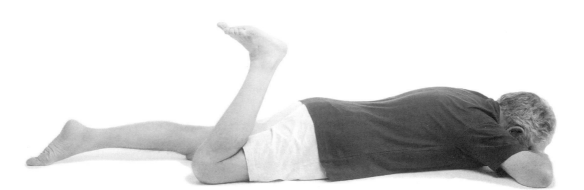

Wall Curls

This is one of the core exercises in any Pilates session.

Aim

To increase awareness of the spine, recognizing any areas which are stiff or 'fused' together. Mobilizing, lengthening and strengthening the muscles which support the spine. You are also working the abdominals, the pelvic floor and the buttocks. What more could you ask from any exercise?

Preparation

You may have a very flat pillow under your head if you are more comfortable with this.

▷ Lie at a distance from a wall, with your pelvis square to it. Feet on the wall in parallel.
▷ Your knees are bent at a right angle, hip-width apart.
▷ Have your arms resting down by your sides, palms down.

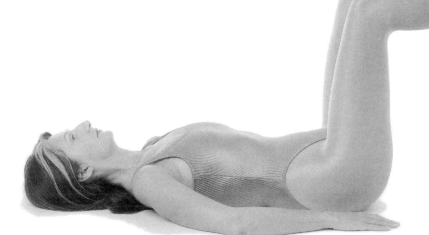

Starting position

Action

▷ Breathe in to prepare.

▷ Breathe out, and draw the lower abdominals back to the spine, lift from the pelvic floor, tighten your buttocks and curl the coccyx (tailbone) just a little off the floor. You will lose the neutral pelvis. You can push into your feet to help.

▷ Breathe in and then out as you lower.

▷ Continue with this, lifting a little more of the spine off the floor each time. *Do not arch the back* (keep in your mind the image of a whippet with its tail between its legs), curl as much of the spine as you can off the floor – but do not go higher than your shoulders.

▷ As you place the spine back down on the floor, do so bone by bone, vertebra by vertebra, separating them. Aim to put three inches between each vertebra. Use your deep abdominals to control your descent. Work out any stiffness.

▷ Repeat five times.

Awareness Points

▷ Keep your abdominals scooped out the whole time.

▷ Please do not come up any higher than you are comfortable with – this is not a balancing trick. The shoulders must stay on the floor.

Up there

Breathing

You are now **relaxed** and hopefully aware of holding on to tension. Already far more aware of your body, we need now to work on learning **good movement practices**.

Mind Body Breathing

Breathing is fundamental to life. It lies on the borderline between the conscious and subconscious and can be influenced by either. Although we will be attempting to 'alter' the way you breathe during the explorations and exercises, it will probably take a long time before your normal breathing patterns are altered.

Ultimately, there are many benefits to breathing more efficiently. The tissues are better nourished, as are the nerves, the glands and the organs. Improved oxygen supply keeps bones, teeth and hair in good condition. The gentle expansion of the ribcage facilitates greater flexibility of the upper body as the muscles between the ribs are exercised regularly. This is also aided by the directions to lengthen up through the spine. Any increase in the distance between vertebrae, with the discs 'plumping up', will improve the suppleness of the ribcage and upper body.

Slow, deep breathing helps to reverse the stress responses in the body by calming the nerves. Breathing deeply while exercising enhances relaxation and allows the mind to relax into the rhythm of the movements.

We have already looked at the mechanics and the reasons behind thoracic/lateral or 'bellow breathing' on page 31. The following explorations and exercises will raise your awareness and control of your breathing. You will notice how subtle changes in the manner and timing of your breath can completely change the way you feel. If you experience light-headedness doing these exercises, take a break. This is simply due to the increase in oxygen and you should quickly return to normal.

CASE STUDY

Elaine, a 39-year-old housewife, was referred by her GP to Piers Chandler for osteopathy. She had been complaining of low back pain – a constant ache for the previous ten years since the birth of her three children (then all under four). It had got to the stage where she was experiencing at least two acute attacks per year and she was starting to feel totally restricted in what she was able to do. The pain was aggravated by gardening and around the time of her period. Previous osteopathy and physiotherapy had helped only temporarily, but Chandler's treatment enabled her to garden again and she became increasingly confident with movement. However, he told her that she should not stop there, so 'reluctantly' she agreed to take up Pilates – everything she had tried before had been so painful.

Elaine began private mat classes with Lynne Robinson, whose Pilates programme began with teaching body awareness, good postural alignment and relaxation skills, as well as correct breathing techniques. Lynne found Elaine's back to be unusually flat and the muscles very weak. As a result, Elaine found back extension too stressful, so concentrated instead on lengthening the back while strengthening the muscles. She also had very poor abdominal strength, so had to learn how to use her core lower abdominals to support her back and create a strong centre from which to work.

The first month was a case of three steps forward, one step back, as her body readjusted to being used in a new way. However, after two months her progress was rapid and quite spectacular. Two years later she is virtually free of pain and also has an enormous sense of well-being. What's more, she is able to perform advanced exercise movements requiring considerable abdominal strength with both grace and ease. As she herself says, 'I now feel that my back has the support it deserves.'

Melting Body

Change the way you feel by changing the way you breathe.

As discussed earlier, exhalation encourages relaxation, whilst inhalation, on the other hand, re-energizes – it 'inspires'. This can be a useful tool and after practising the following exercise and experiencing the changes that occur, you will be able to apply this principle in everyday life.

Preparation

▷ Retreat into a quiet corner and make sure that you will not be interrupted for about fifteen minutes.

▷ You can either adopt the Relaxation Position or support your raised legs by placing a rolled-up duvet underneath, keeping your legs apart, knees bent.

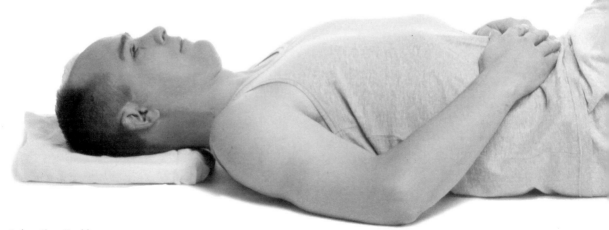

Relaxation Position

Action

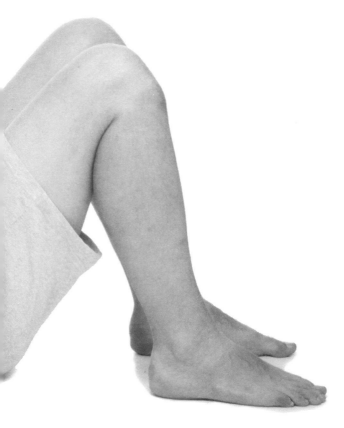

▷ Focus on your breath. Initially you might like to encourage thoracic breathing by placing your hands on the lower ribcage. With the floor as a guide you can more easily feel the widening of your ribcage.

▷ Breathe in through your nose, breathe out through your mouth.

▷ As in the Relaxation Position, we start from the feet and work our way to the top. Focus on your feet and count to five on your out-breath. Inhale on the count of 'three'.

▷ It is as if the out-breath is 'melting' any muscular tension that you discover in your feet.

▷ Repeat three times, gently and steadily exhaling. During inhalation, imagine that rejuvenating energy is entering and filling your body.

▷ After the feet, shift your focus to your ankles, calves, knees, thighs and so on. A longer exhalation than inhalation helps to calm the nervous system and the mind and induces a powerful state of relaxation.

▷ Once you have reached the head, be aware of how you feel.

▷ Stay with this way of breathing for a few moments, then you will change the pattern. Increase inhalation to the count of five, and decrease exhalation to the count of three.

▷ Repeat three times on each part of the body, and let inhalation re-energize each part. Gradually work your way down towards the feet.

▷ Depending on the time of day, you might also stay with one type of breathing. If you are exercising last thing at night, continued exhalation can aid relaxation before sleep. If first thing in the morning, continued inhalation can increase energy and help you to get out of bed!

▷ You might also consider focusing on your breath during the day to either calm your nerves or increase your energy, as required.

Beach Ball Hamstrings

Aim

To lengthen the back, gently stretching the spine. To stretch the hamstring muscles at the back of your legs.

These are very calming exercises, so approach them gently. The aim is not to take your head down on to your knee, but rather to lengthen out the spine. You will feel quite a stretch in the hamstrings, even though you are not going right down on to your leg.

Preparation

▷ Sit with your legs out in front of you. Make sure that you are sitting squarely and not twisting in the pelvis – you can line yourself up with the wall, if you wish.

▷ Bend the left knee and place the sole of the foot on the inside of the right knee.

▷ Your right leg is straight, the kneecap facing directly up to the ceiling – do not let it roll in or out. Your right knee is soft and not locked back, your foot is relaxed. Keep your left hip aligned.

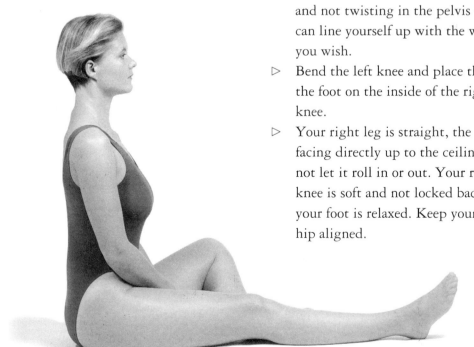

Starting position

Action

▷ Breathe in to prepare, and lengthen up through the spine.

▷ Breathe out, draw the navel to the spine, and lift up out of your pelvis and up and over an imaginary beach ball, so that you are coming up and over, directing in front of you.

▷ Take ten slow breaths, relaxing into the position. Check that your shoulders stay down into your back. Your neck is long, the top of your head lengthening away towards your foot. Your elbows are open and relaxed.

▷ Slowly come back up into an upright position.

▷ Repeat on the other side.

Awareness Points

▷ Try to keep the beach ball image to prevent you from simply collapsing.

▷ Stay aware of the position of your shoulderblades as they must stay down into your back.

▷ Keep central, do not twist to one side.

Full position

Triceps Stretch

Aim

To open the upper body, stretching the triceps and pectoral muscles.

You may find that your hands do not meet, in which case you can use a scarf to help bring them closer together. Most people have about a ten per cent size difference between their right and left sides.

Preparation

Stand or sit, with your pelvis in neutral. Have one hand on the back of your head, at the top of the spine, the other hand at the base of the spine.

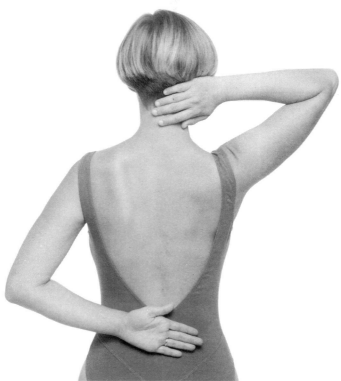

Starting position

Action

▷ Breathe in to prepare and lengthen up through the spine.

▷ Breathe out and begin to trace the spine with your fingers, so that your two hands meet.

▷ Take a couple of deep breaths in this position, taking advantage of the openness of your chest. Keep your head central, your ribs wide.

▷ On your next out-breath, slowly trace the spine again as you take the arms back to the starting position and then down by your side.

▷ Repeat with the other side, doing three to each side.

Awareness Points

▷ The top of your head should stay central and lengthening up – try not to twist or turn it to one side or drop forward.

▷ Just keep an eye out that you do not arch your back to help your hands meet. The pelvis must stay in neutral!

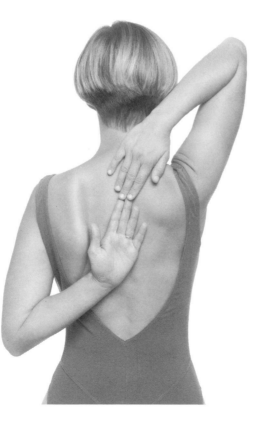

Full position

Curl Ups

Aim

▷ To use the breath to aid movement.
▷ To strengthen the abdominals.
▷ To learn to curl the upper body while keeping the navel pulled back to the spine.
▷ To minimize the use of the neck muscles.
▷ To use the spine as a wheel.

Note

If you have neck problems please do not attempt this exercise.

Preparation

▷ Lie on your back.
▷ Have your feet hip-width apart and in parallel.
▷ Before you start the exercise, just allow your head to gently roll from side to side, which will release the neck.
▷ Then, place one hand on the side of your head, the other on your lower abdomen. This is to check that your stomach does not pop up.

Action

▷ Breathe in to prepare.
▷ As you start to breathe out, hollow out the lower abdominals.
▷ Then, soften your breastbone and curl up, breaking from the breastbone. Keep a small gap under your chin, let your ribs close down and the tailbone also stays down, lengthening away from you. Only go as far as you can while keeping your stomach hollowed out. The minute your stomach begins to pop up, curl back down. Do not pull on the neck!
▷ Breathe in as you slowly curl back down.
▷ Open the elbow back to the floor each time.
▷ Repeat five times, then change hands and do five more.
▷ When you have mastered keeping the stomach hollowed out, you may place

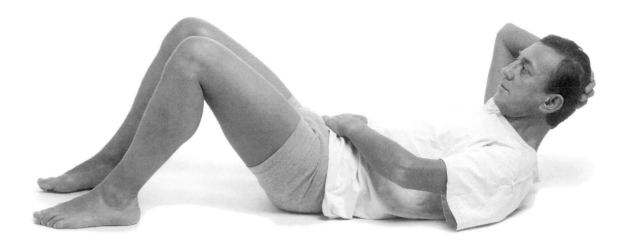

Full position

both hands behind your head for support. Open the elbows out and down at the end of each curl up.

▷ Don't forget to open out the elbows when you have completed each curl up, as it will help to discourage round shoulders.

Awareness Points

▷ Keep the lower abdominals hollowed out as you come up.

▷ Keep your neck released, the shoulders relaxed, a gap under your chin.

▷ Keep your tailbone on the floor, lengthening away from you. Try not to tighten around your hip joints. The front of the pelvis keeps its length.

▷ Do not pull on your head or neck.

▷ Stop if you feel any strain in the neck.

Oblique Curl Ups

Aim

To work the oblique stomach muscles, without stressing the neck and still maintaining the curling action of the spine. To keep a sense of openness in the upper body.

Preparation

▷ Lie with the knees bent, hip-width apart and in parallel.

▷ Bend your left knee and place the ankle to rest just above the right knee, with the left knee then opening.

▷ Place your left hand behind your left thigh, the elbow open.

▷ Your right hand can be placed on the side of your head.

▷ Keep the hip bones in line.

Action

▷ Breathe in to prepare.

▷ Breathe out, hollow navel to spine, and curl up, breaking from the breastbone as above.

Full position

▷ Bring your right shoulder across towards your left knee. The elbow stays back as it is the shoulder which moves forward. Your stomach must stay hollow.

▷ Breathe in and lower.

▷ Repeat five times, and then change sides.

Awareness Points

▷ Keep the upper body open and the neck released.

▷ The pelvis stays neutral and square, and the elbows back.

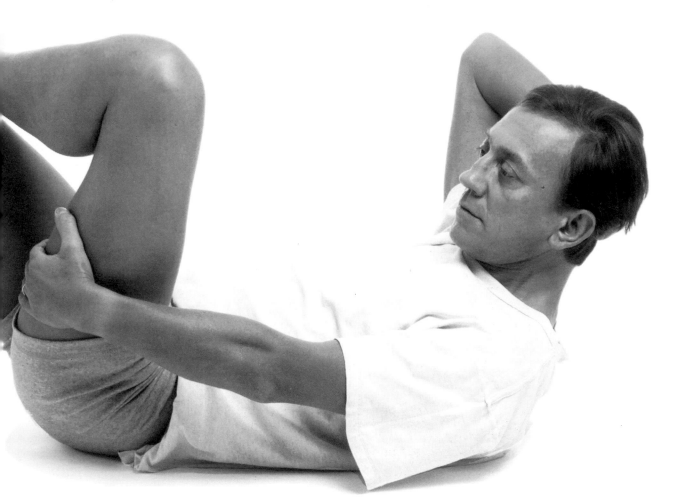

Curl Ups with a Scarf

With traditional sit-ups the movement is often led by the head and neck which can stress the neck. This exercise helps to reinforce the correct way to curl up – breaking from the breastbone and sternum, whilst keeping the neck soft and the upper body open.

Aim

To strengthen the abdominals without compromising the neck. To co-ordinate the breath with movement.

Preparation

You will need a scarf or pole.

Lie on your back, holding the scarf in your hands above your head. Your hands should be about a metre apart, the wrists in line, the elbows bent, the shoulders soft and open.

Action

▷ Breathe in to prepare.
▷ Breathe out, draw the lower abdominals back to the spine, and bring the knees on to your chest, one at a time.

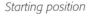

Starting position

- ▷ Breathe in and bring the scarf to the level of your chest, keeping the arms long and the elbows bent and open.
- ▷ Breathe out, drawing the lower abdominals firmly back to your spine and softening your neck and chest. Hinge up from the breastbone, the ribs close down and together. Your arms come down along your sides, elbows open, shoulderblades down into your back.
- ▷ Breathe in as you slowly curl back down.
- ▷ Repeat ten times.

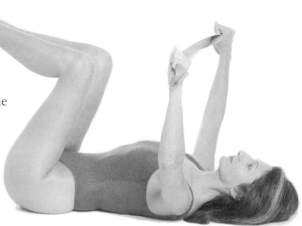

Bring the scarf to the level of your chest

Awareness Points

- ▷ As both your arms and legs are off the floor, you need to have your back firmly anchored. You do not need to keep the pelvis in neutral here, although you should keep a sense of lengthening the pelvis.
- ▷ Be sure that you only start to raise your head when the scarf is above your nose.
- ▷ The shoulderblades stay open and down into your back.

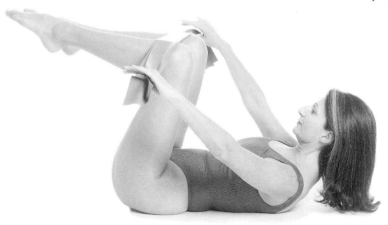

Full position

Twister

Many people hurt their backs in the car when twisting around to reverse or to get something off the back seat. If you take a moment, breathe and lengthen, create a strong centre and then turn, you will be much less likely to do yourself a mischief.

It is interesting to note how the breath can help or hinder a movement.

When the Pilates Method was originally taught, rotation of the spine, like the twisting here, was always done on the out-breath, but recently we have been experimenting with rotating on the in-breath and have found that it actually enhances the movement.

We have given you both options here. We recommend twisting on the in-breath only if you are fully fit. If you have a back problem, use the chair position and twist with the out-breath as it reinforces the stabilizing muscles and will give you more protection.

Please avoid this exercise if you have a disc-related injury.

Aim

Using the breath, to learn to lengthen before you twist. To work the muscles which run the length of the spine. To work the waist.

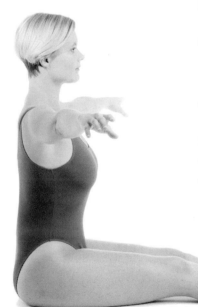

Starting position

Preparation

Sit long-legged. You may like to place a rolled-up towel under your buttocks to help tip yourself forward (this will bring the pelvis into line). If this is still too uncomfortable for you, or if you are having difficulty keeping the spine in neutral, then try sitting on a chair.

Action

▷ Breathe in to prepare and lengthen up through the spine, raising your arms to shoulder height, taking care to keep your neck relaxed.

▷ Breathe out, navel to spine and, lengthening upwards, turn to look over your shoulder – only as far as you are comfortable. Your arms stay in line with each other, like aeroplane wings. Keep the pelvis still and square.

▷ Breathe in and lengthen, the shoulderblades staying down into your back.

▷ Return to centre.

▷ Repeat three times to each side.

Working on the Inhalation

As mentioned above you may also try this exercise, rotating on the in-breath as follows:

▷ Breathe in to prepare and lengthen up through the spine.

▷ Breathe out, navel to spine.

▷ Breathe in, lengthening up through the top of your head and twist around, turning to look over your shoulder – only as far as you are comfortable. Your arms stay in line with each other, like aeroplane wings.

▷ Breathe out, navel to spine, and return to centre.

▷ Repeat three times to each side.

Chair Twist

An alternative

If sitting for a long period or holding your arms out is difficult for you, then try the following version:

Preparation

Sit on straight-backed chair, your feet firmly planted on the floor, hip-width apart. The knees are at right angles. Fold your arms in front of you, in line with your chest.

Action

▷ Breathe in and lengthen up through the spine.

▷ Breathe out, navel to spine, and turn to the right as far as you can, keeping the pelvis square on the chair and forward facing. Your arms stay at chest height.

▷ Breathe in and, lengthening upwards, return to the front.

▷ Repeat three times in each direction.

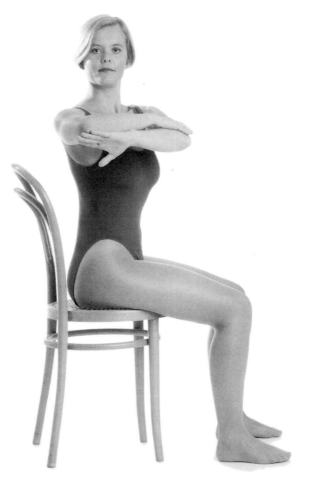

Full position

CASE STUDY

Jenny, aged 38, is an administrator. She underwent osteopathy with Piers Chandler after two years of upper back and shoulder pain following a road traffic accident three years earlier. Jenny has a scoliosis 'S'-shape (see page 29), with a high left shoulder and high right hip and, while the osteopath's treatment helped, he felt she needed to try 'whole body exercise'.

So Jenny joined a group mat work Pilates class. The sessions included exercises to improve body awareness, alignment, relaxation, breathing, core stability, strength and flexibility. Before long, she felt much improved abdominal strength and a greater range of movement. On a return visit to her osteopath, she was told that her improved posture had made her taller and her back broader!

The overall postural programme helped with her scoliosis and additional remedial exercises for stretching and mobilizing her upper body and shoulders combined with work to stabilize her scapulae and strengthen the lower trapezius. She also used light weights to help build her strength.

Jenny found it easy to fit Pilates into her life: the classes were enjoyable and relaxing, and she was able to follow the routine easily at home. At the time of writing, she had only needed to visit the osteopath once in the previous eighteen months, and her general level of fitness had dramatically improved.

Spine Curls with Breath

This is a variation of the Wall Curls (see page 86) but uses the breath. Notice how by timing the movement of the arms with the breath, the whole direction of the exercise changes.

Preparation

▷ Lie on your back with your knees bent, your feet about twenty centimetres from your buttocks.

▷ Your feet should be hip-width apart and parallel. Plant them firmly onto the floor.

▷ Leave the arms by your side, palms down.

Action

▷ Breathe in to prepare.

▷ Breathe out and hollow out the lower abdominal muscles down towards the spine, engaging the muscles of the pelvic floor and the buttocks.

▷ Slowly and carefully, lift just the base of your spine (the coccyx, or tailbone) off the floor – you will lose the neutral pelvis position.

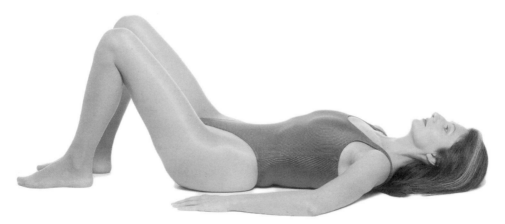

Starting position

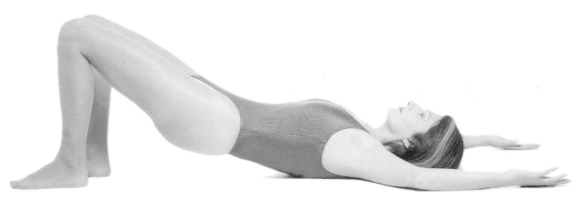

Take your arms above your head as you breathe in

▷ Breathe in, and breathe out as you lower and lengthen the spine back on to the floor.

▷ Repeat, lifting a little more of the spine off the floor each time. As you lower, put down each part of the spine in sequence – bone by bone, aiming to put three inches between each vertebra – the back of the ribs, the waist, the small of the back, the tailbone. *Only when this is down* do you lower and release the buttocks. Use the lower abdominals throughout.

▷ When you have lifted the spine as high as it can comfortably come off the floor without arching, on your next in-breath you take the arms above your head to touch the floor behind. Keep them open and wide, the elbows soft.

▷ Breathe out and, bone by bone, lengthen the spine down on the floor, stretching the tailbone away from the top of your head.

▷ When the tailbone 'lands', breathe in again, and bring your arms down by your side.

▷ Repeat five times, timing the breath with the arm movements. Remember: When you have finished the exercise gently stretch out your hip flexors (see next exercise).

Breathing

▷ Breathe out as you raise the spine.
▷ Breathe in whilst the spine is raised, taking the arms behind you.
▷ Breathe out as you slowly lower it.

Awareness Points

▷ Please do not allow the back to arch. Keep the tailbone tucked under like a whippet who's just been ticked off.
▷ Keep your feet parallel, don't let them roll in or out. The weight should stay evenly balanced.
▷ Remember to peel the vertebrae off bone by bone, separating them.
▷ Check your neck – don't let it arch back, keep it long and released.

Hip Flexor Stretch

Aim

To gently stretch the hip flexors, which are inclined to shorten after periods of prolonged sitting.

Action

▷ Breathe in to prepare.

▷ Breathe out, hollow out the lower abdominals, navel to spine, and –

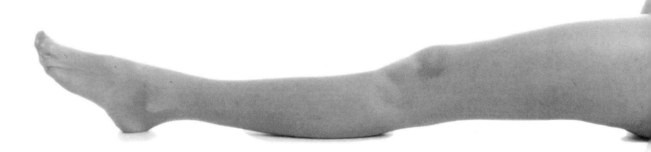

keeping that sense of hollowness in the pelvis – hinge the right knee up to your chest, dropping the thigh bone down into the hip joint.

Women – Bring the knee very slightly towards your right shoulder.

Men – keep the knee in line with your chest.

▷ Breathe in as you clasp the right leg below the knee, or behind the lower part of the thigh, if you have joint problems.

▷ Holding on to the leg, breathe out as you extend the left leg along the floor. If your lower back arches, bend the left knee back up again a little.

▷ Take a couple of breaths to allow the muscle to stretch out.

▷ Breathe in as you slide the left leg back up to the starting position.

▷ Breathe out as you lower the right bent knee to the floor, keeping the abdominals engaged and a sense of hollowness in the abdomen.

▷ Repeat twice on each side.

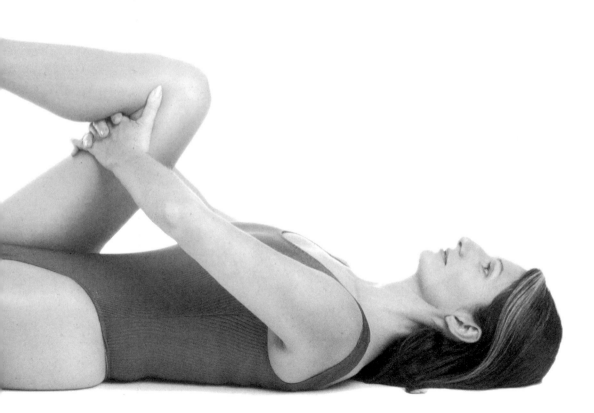

Use of Centre

The creation of a 'girdle of strength' from which to work was one of the main goals of **Joseph Pilates'** fitness programme. Pilates builds strength from within by teaching you to use your **stabilizing muscles**.

Mind Body – Use of Centre

The exercises in this chapter follow on from the preliminary 'navel to spine' work on page 33.

There are other reasons, however, why we work from the centre of the body. It is also the centre of balance, the centre of gravity, and the centre of control.

The body has three main 'weights':

▷ The Head
▷ The Ribcage (Thorax)
▷ The Pelvis

Notice how they are positioned over each other and around a vertical plumbline. Our centre of gravity is balanced over the base of our support, that is, our feet.

If you take a cross-section of the lower body, cutting yourself at the centre, this is what you would see:

The Head

The Ribcage

The Pelvis

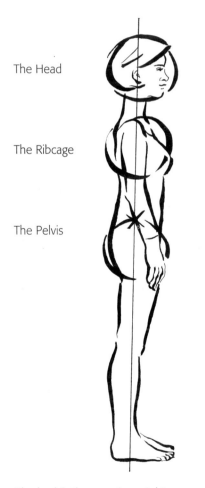

The body's three main weights

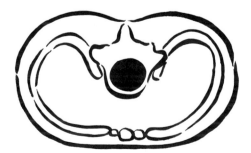

Cross-section

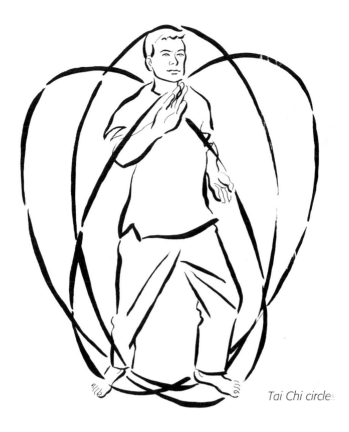

Tai Chi circle

Notice the thickness of the lumbar vertebrae. The front of the spine is, in fact, at the centre of your body, not the at the back. The centre of gravity lies just behind the navel, in front of the spine, by the third or fourth lumbar vertebra. A large, muscle-controlling nerve centre is also located here.

It is no wonder, therefore, that the concept of 'the centre' has been influential for over two thousand years in the Far East, where it is referred to as the 'Hara'. It is believed that this centre of the body's strength is located in the abdominal area. In anatomical terms we would define the *Hara* as the area between the pelvic bone and the ribcage. This part of our body contains most of our vital organs, digestive and reproductive functions taking place here. Because food is digested in this area, so releasing energy, we can easily recognize the importance of the *Hara.*

The *Hara* is also believed to play an important role in terms of emotions. When you are really upset, all your tension is concentrated in that area and the same applies for true laughter, also known as a belly laugh. Being in touch with your *Hara* will also have a positive effect on your emotions.

The Chinese art of T'ai Chi Ch'uan was the forerunner of all the eastern martial arts, such as karate, jujitsu and aikido. As one practices T'ai Chi, very much a mind body discipline, one is encouraged to feel the flow of energy from the centre or '*tant'tien*'.

Lengthening away from the Centre

We are following on here from where we left off in Chapter 3 concerning the basic rules for good body use. Now, we are aiming to apply and maintain our core stability while we move our limbs. It looks easy, but requires great control to be correctly executed.

Aim

To maintain a strong centre – your 'core stability' – while moving the limbs.

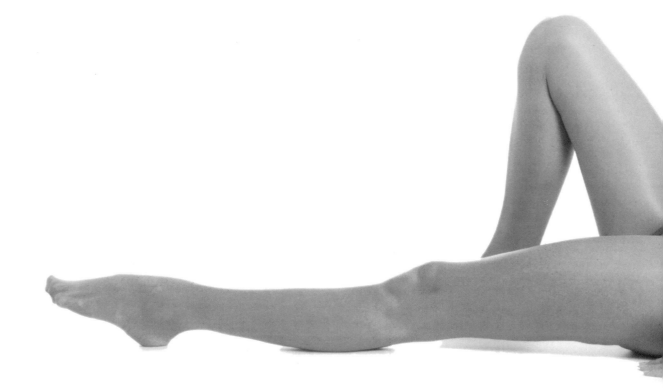

Slide the leg away

Preparation

Adopt the Relaxation Position. Check that your pelvis is in neutral, tailbone down and lengthening away.

Action

▷ Breathe in to prepare.
▷ Breathe out completely, draw the lower abdominals back to the spine (navel to spine), and slide one leg away along the floor, keeping the lower abdominals engaged and the pelvis still, stable, and in neutral.
▷ Breathe into your lower ribcage while you return the leg to the bent position, trying to keep the stomach hollow.
▷ Repeat five times with each leg.

Awareness Points

▷ Remember to keep the leg on the floor.
▷ Your pelvis remains as still as possible.

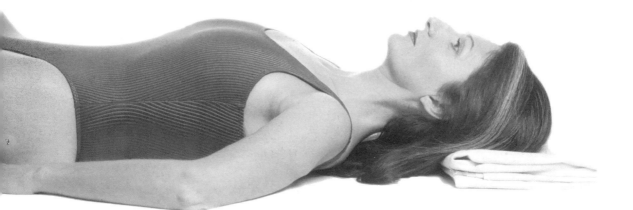

Adding the Arms

Aim

To practice moving the arms while stabilizing the trunk. To encourage the correct use of the shoulder muscles.

Preparation

Relaxation Position, as in previous exercise, but take your arms down by your sides, palms down.

Arm above head

Action

▷ Breathe in wide into your lower ribcage to prepare.

▷ Breathe out, navel to spine, and take one arm back to touch the floor behind. Do not force it – keep the elbow soft and open. The shoulderblade stays down into your back. The ribs stay calm.

▷ Breathe in as you return the arm to your side.

▷ Repeat with the other arm. Practice five times on each arm.

Note

Not everyone can touch the floor behind without arching the upper back, so do not strain. It is better to keep the back down than force the arm.

Now is the time to be more adventurous. In the next exercise we will use opposite arms and legs.

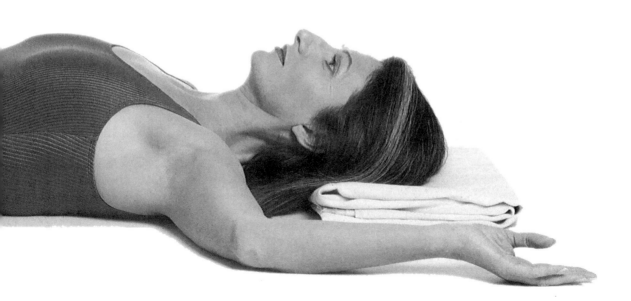

Co-ordinating Arms and Legs (Starfish)

Action

▷ Breathe in to prepare.

▷ Breathe out, hollow 'navel to spine' and slide the right leg away along the floor and take the left arm above you in a backstroke movement and touch the floor behind, if you can. Think of a starfish. Keep the pelvis completely neutral, stable and still and the stomach muscles engaged. Keep a sense of width and openness in the upper body and shoulders, and try to keep the shoulderblades down into your back.

▷ Breathe in, navel still to spine, and return the limbs to the starting position.

▷ Repeat five times, alternating arms and legs.

These may not seen like difficult movements but to do them properly takes great concentration and skill.

Awareness Points

▷ No wobbling, twisting, dipping, tucking, tilting, listing . . . keep stable!

▷ Keep the lower abdominals firmly engaged.

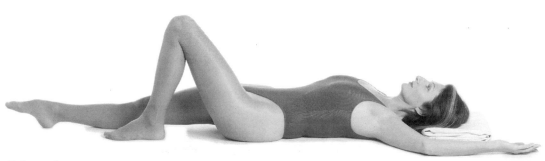

Full stretch

Full Body Stretch

This is wonderful after Curl Ups. You must be able to do the previous exercises without wobbling the pelvis before progressing to this stretch. We do not recommend it for those of you with back problems. You should continue instead with the Co-ordinating Arms and Legs Stretch.

Aim

To feel the use of centre while enjoying a full body stretch.

Preparation

Relaxation Position, as in previous exercise.

Action

▷ Breathe in to prepare.
▷ Breathe out, create a strong centre by hollowing 'navel to spine' and then stretch both arms and legs away from you, so that you are 'reaching' your fingers away from your toes. Think yourself 'thin' and strong in the centre.
▷ Breathe in and bring both arms back down to your side.
▷ Breathe out and bend the knees back one at a time to the bent position. Keep the centre strong.
▷ Repeat five times.

Awareness Points

If you feel that you are losing your neutral pelvis, go back to practising with Co-ordinating Arms and Legs for a little while longer.

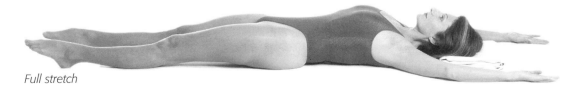

Full stretch

Chalk Circle

In this exercise you are going to imagine that you are holding a piece of chalk in your top hand, and draw a chalk circle on the floor. If your upper body is tight and your shoulders stiff, you will find it uncomfortable at first and you may not be able to keep in touch with the floor. Move within your limits, don't push yourself too far, keep the elbow bent.

As you do this exercise more often the upper body opens out and it feels wonderful.

Please avoid this exercise if you have a disc-related injury.

Preparation

▷ Lie on your side with a pillow under your head – a bed pillow is perfect.
▷ Have your back in a straight line but curl your knees up to hip level.
▷ Extend your arms in front of you, in line with your shoulders, palms together.

Aim

To open the upper body, stretching the tight muscles (pectorals and anterior deltoids) using the centre. To help release tension.

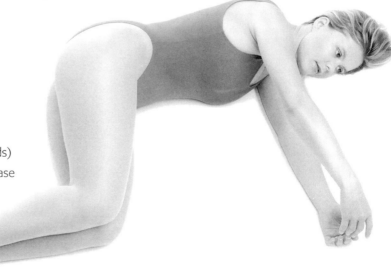

Starting position

Action

▷ Breathe in to prepare.

▷ Breathe out, create a strong centre and, reaching the top arm beyond the lower arm, take your hand above you over your head. Allow your head to follow the movement of the shoulders. The knees stay together and the centre strong but now breathe normally.

▷ Reach your hand right around as if you are drawing the circle on the floor. It will pass behind you, over your buttocks and back up to join the other hand.

▷ Repeat five times on each side.

Awareness Points

▷ Please do not forget to move your head as well.

▷ Keep your knees together on the floor.

▷ Keep your hips in line, one directly over the other.

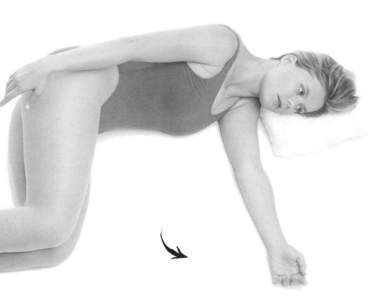

Side Rolls

Aim

To learn how to initiate movement from the centre. To stretch the muscles along the spine.

Please avoid this exercise if you have a disc-related injury.

Preparation

▷ Lie on your back, your head on a small, flat, firm pillow.

▷ Your feet should be parallel on the floor, hip-width apart.

▷ Your arms are down by your sides away from the body, palms down.

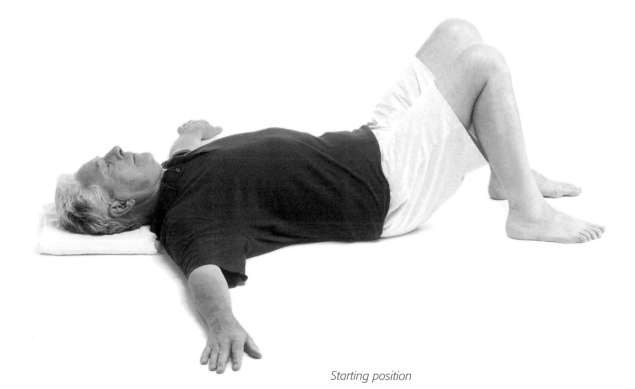

Starting position

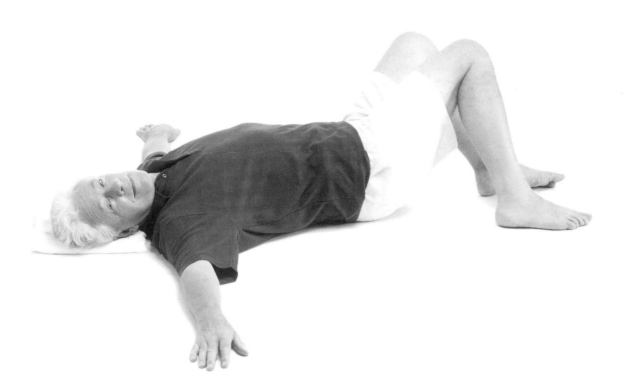

Action

▷ Breathe in to prepare.

▷ Breathe out, navel to spine, and roll your head in one direction, your knees in the other. Only go as far as you can, keeping your opposite shoulder down on the floor.

▷ Breathe in, keeping the stomach hollow.

▷ Breathe out, navel to spine, and bring the knees back to centre.

▷ Repeat five times each way.

Awareness Points

Remember to keep the opposite shoulderblade down on the floor.

Pelvic Roll Backs

Aim

To co-ordinate the breath with the use of centre and movement of the spine. To strengthen the deep abdominals.

This is a powerful stomach muscle exercise, so approach with caution. We suggest that you roll back just a little to begin with and then further as you are more comfortable with the movement.

Please avoid this exercise if you have a disc-related injury or lumbar-sacral problems.

Preparation

▷ Sit on the floor, knees bent, feet parallel and hip-width apart.

▷ Hold your legs behind the thighs, just above the back of the knees.

▷ Plant your feet well onto the floor. Remember the triangle – base of the big toe, base of the small toe, centre of the heel, keep the weight even on these three points.

Action

▷ Breathe in to prepare and lengthen up through the spine.

▷ Breathe out, hollow out the lower abdominals and, keeping them hollow, curl back on to your tailbone, rounding your lower back and rotating the pelvis – the pubic bone stays fixed, the front of the pelvis long and not scrunched up.

Your upper body is curled but not collapsed, keep the elbows open, the neck soft, the shoulderblades down into your back.

Starting position

▷ Breathe in, navel to spine still, and uncurl the spine to an upright position. The shoulders stay relaxed and down.

Rolled Back

▷ Now, imagining that there is a cord attached to your breastbone, pulling forward and up, open the chest towards the ceiling. Breathe out, open the chest and take your head back just a little to look at the top corner of the room where the wall meets the ceiling – *do not take it back any further*. The neck stays long.

▷ Breathe in and come upright again.

Open chest

▷ Repeat five times.

Awareness Points

▷ Everyone tends to roll their feet outwards. Keep them firmly planted, the big toes anchored onto the floor.

▷ Do not drop or throw your head back or you will overextend your neck. It is a very small subtle movement, just lengthening the neck gently.

Grounding

It was **Sir Isaac Newton** who first discovered that for every action there is an equal and opposing reaction. **Gravity** is one of the great **forces of nature**, making things fall and keeping the planets in their orbits.

Grounding

Everything we do is affected by gravity. We are so accustomed to it that our bones grow weaker without it, which is what happens when astronauts spend any length of time in space. The force of gravity acts to pull everything towards the centre of the earth, but because the earth is compact, when gravity pulls an object down to the ground, the ground in turn, resists. This resistance takes the form of a bounce, a force upward, opposite and equal to the downward force. Our bodies are subject to this constant action and reaction, up and down, keeping the body both balanced and upright, the muscles working constantly. This is why we need to maintain our centre of gravity, and also why we need to 'ground' ourselves.

In our society a lot of emphasis is placed upon intellectual achievement, to the extent that mental ability seems to be rated higher than any physical or manual talents. This over-emphasis on intellectual skills will quite often result in an energy imbalance, for continued mental stimulation 'draws' a lot of energy towards the head, leaving the body in a general state of imbalance.

Working on your own feet can bring back that balance, drawing energy back to the feet. These provide our base of support and our connection to the ground, the earth. The feet contain many nerve endings for sensing and responding – they inform us of the stability of our base. Our feet act as shock absorbers, give us stability and mobility and spread the bodyweight to the ground.

Yet we still mistreat our feet considerably, frequently by wearing shoes that are too tight or high-heeled. This results in a very narrowed foot and, therefore, a narrow-based platform for the whole of our body. These problems can be exacerbated by our surroundings; for example flat concrete surfaces also decrease the sensitivity of our feet and result in restricted ankle mobility.

The explorations and exercises in this chapter will focus your attention on the sound foundation of your feet! We hope they will help you to:

▷ Get in touch with your feet
▷ Become aware of the effect of the feet on the rest of your body
▷ Increase the mobility in your feet
▷ Increase strength in, especially, the arch of the foot
▷ Correct any misalignments such as rolling in and rolling out.

CASE STUDY

Charles, a businessman in his thirties, came to the Pilates studio after his wife had booked him in. He had suffered years of backache, and couldn't even perform simple tasks, like picking things up off the floor. He felt generally very unfit, but having been previously bullied at a gym he was quite apprehensive about attending a session.

Charles needed lots of encouragement and deep abdominal work to stabilize his back. He came twice a week, and the improvement was very encouraging from day one. After this strengthening work, he moved on to more weight-bearing exercises, and soon noted a vast improvement of his overall muscle tone. His sedentary lifestyle made stretching as well as strengthening a very important part of his programme.

In his own words, 'My general energy level has increased, and I find I don't fall asleep on the sofa when I get home at night. My flexibility has also increased – just the other day I noticed how I was able to pick up my kids' toys from the floor without any trouble!'

Foot Massage

You can do this as often as you like, but it is especially beneficial after long periods of standing, walking or driving.

Note

Do not do this if your foot is injured in any way – please consult your specialist first.

Aim

To stimulate the nerve endings in your foot and increase circulation, mobility, awareness and flexibility.

Preparation

▷ Wash your feet with some warm water in order to increase the circulation and soften the skin.

▷ Sit comfortably in your favourite chair with plenty of cushions to support your back.

▷ Depending on the range of movement in your hip joint, sit cross-legged and place one foot on the opposite thigh. Don't worry if you cannot do this, as only a few people are able to do so whilst leaving the rest of the body relaxed.

▷ Draw one leg up, the knee towards your chest, keeping the leg in parallel. This way you can easily reach the back of the foot and the sole with the fingers.

▷ Work with a partner, who sits on the floor in front of you while supporting your knee with cushions.

Action

▷ Stroke the whole of the foot with a flat, relaxed hand, not forgetting to include the ankles. You might want to use a little moisturising lotion to glide more easily. When working with a partner, use a firm but soft touch to help them relax, yet to reassure them at the same time.

▷ Circle one toe at a time gently in its socket.

▷ Pinch the skin between the toes with the thumb and the index finger.

▷ With two to three fingers, circle all over the foot – avoid the ankles if you or your partner are pregnant or are trying to conceive.

▷ Press with your thumbs on the bottom of your foot (this might be a little painful, especially around the instep of your foot). You should do whatever feels good so, when you are working with a partner, always ask for their comments and guidance.

Standing Like a Tree

This exercise has it roots in Chi Kung.

These images will help you to prepare for the following exploration:

▷ Trees are exposed to the elements.
▷ They reach deep into the soil with their roots.
▷ They reach towards the light.
▷ They take strength from the earth, from water and rain, from the sun, from the air and from the space that surrounds them.

Preparation

Use the guidelines on page 54 (Standing).

Action

▷ Your weight is evenly distributed between your left and right foot. These 'roots' sink deep into the earth, like those of a tree.

　From below your kneecaps, your roots extend downwards.

　From your knees upwards, you rise

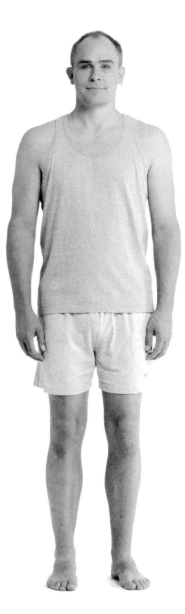

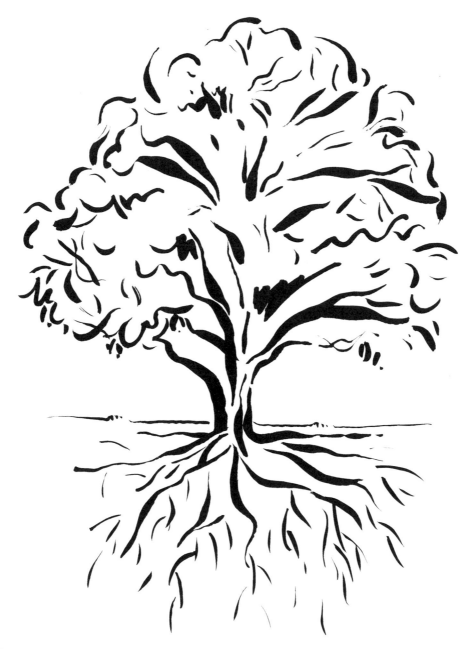

like a tree – lengthening your spine, resting calmly between the earth and the sky.

▷ On your next out-breath, let any unnecessary tension that you discover flow down towards your feet, into the imaginary roots and, from there, into the ground.

▷ On your next in-breath draw rejuvenating energy from the earth, into the imaginary roots, filling the whole of your body.

Grounding while Sitting

The following exercise is particularly useful if you spend a lot of your time sitting. Our bodies are simply not designed to sit for long periods. It is extremely difficult to keep the body in good alignment whilst carrying out small range movements, such as typing or writing. Often the kind of chair we sit on is blamed for encouraging 'slouched' posture. Some chairs are better than others, but you can still sit badly in the most expensive, ergonomically designed chair!

Remaining grounded while sitting is very important, especially as most of the activity is focusing around the upper body, resulting in over-tension of the body.

Preparation

▷ Sit with your legs hip-width apart, toes parallel.

▷ Sit close to the edge of the chair, do not rest against the back of the chair!

▷ Be aware of your sitting bones. You can feel them when you 'wiggle' your bottom from cheek to cheek. This is the part of your pelvis you should be sitting on, not the tail of your spine, the coccyx.

▷ Let your hands rest on your thighs.

▷ Maintain a neutral pelvis and spine while sitting.

▷ Release your neck muscles and let the back lengthen.

Action

▷ Be aware of your feet, make them wide, let them melt into the floor.

▷ Check that you are not holding unnecessary tension in your hip joint by gently moving your knees from side to side.

▷ Release the neck muscles by gently nodding your head.

▷ Imagine that the head is releasing upwards and, as a result, the spine is becoming longer with the distance between the vertebrae increasing.

▷ Release any tension in your arms and feel how they become lighter.

▷ Let the feet soften and 'send' the heels into the ground. You can ask a friend to help you by putting their hands on your feet.

Tennis Ball Massage

The following exploration can be done instead of the Foot Massage.

Nerve endings in the feet are stimulated during this exploration and indirectly have both a relaxing and stimulating effect on the rest of the body. It is especially interesting to massage one foot first and to observe any changes that occur in the same half of the body.

This exploration is great after wearing tight shoes over a long period of time. Your feet will come alive and your ankles will be mobilized.

Preparation

▷   Stand with your feet fairly close together, making sure you balance the body weights and are not holding any tensions. Take special care to release your knees.

▷   Place a tennis ball or an orange on the floor.

Action

▷   Transfer your weight on to your right leg, still lengthening your back.

▷   Place your left foot on the ball or orange.

▷   Gently roll the ball under the sole of your foot, making sure you reach all the areas. Try putting more weight on to the foot which is rolling over the ball – be careful if you are using an orange as you might end up standing in a pool of orange juice!

▷   After 3–4 minutes, place the foot back on the floor and balance your weight evenly between the feet. Take note of any changes that have occurred in the left side of your body. Sometimes it helps to close your eyes to focus fully inside the body.

▷   To make your other side feel the same, repeat the sequence with the right foot.

Ankle Circles

The muscles on the outer side of the ankle tend to be weak, which is why so many of us are prone to sprained ankles as you 'roll over' on the outside. This exercise is great for strengthening them.

It also demonstrates clearly that it is far more difficult to execute an exercise slowly than quickly. Follow the instructions below, but when you have finished, just try to do the exercise quickly … and note the difference!

Aim

▷ To free the ankle joint, increasing its mobility.
▷ To work the muscles, ligaments and tendons surrounding the ankle joint.
▷ To work the calf muscles.

Preparation

▷ Lie on your back in the Relaxation Position.
▷ Bend one knee up and put both hands just behind the knee, with your thumbs coming round in front of it – this is so that you can feel if your leg is moving.

Action

▷ Slowly start to circle the foot around very, very slowly and, taking it as far as you can, go to the maximum. The leg should stay completely still, the movement coming totally from the ankle joint. Do not just wiggle your toes around.
▷ Do five circles each way.

Awareness Points

▷ What about the rest of your body when you did this?
▷ What was happening to your jaw and mouth?
▷ What about the other leg – did it stay in line with your hip?

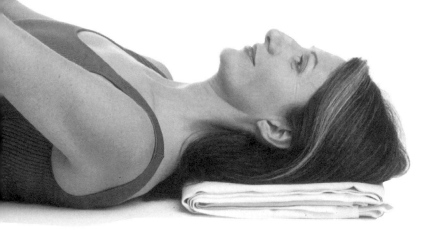

Cherry Picking

Aim

To learn to use all the muscles in the foot, ankle and calves. To increase the arches of the foot.

Preparation

▷ Lie on your back in the Relaxation Position.
▷ Bend one knee up and put your hand just behind the knee, with your thumbs coming round in front of it – this is so that you can feel if your leg is moving.
▷ Soften your elbows and open your chest.

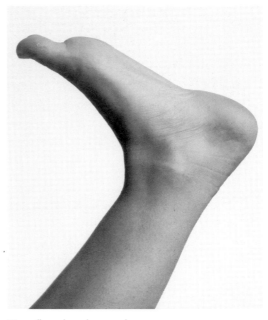

Toes flexed and spread

Action

▷ Keeping your heel still and in line with your knees and hips, flex the foot towards your face, then flex the toes towards your face and spread them as wide as possible.

▷ Keeping them flexed, push through the ball of your foot as you straighten the foot, keeping the heel still.
▷ Now imagine that a cherry tree is there. Pick a cherry by clasping it with the toes.
▷ Keeping the prized cherry firmly clasped in your toes, flex the foot back towards your face.

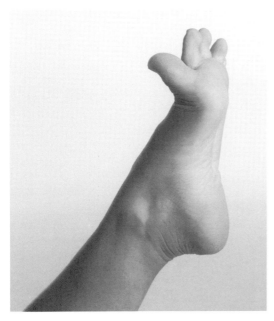

Toes flexed, foot pointing

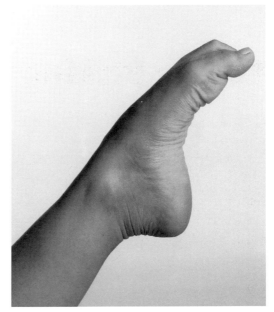

Cherry picked and on way back

▷ Drop the cherry into an imaginary basket and let go of the foot.

▷ Collect five cherries with each foot!

Awareness Points

Did you screw your face up in agony?

Tennis Balls

An exercise like this works on all parts of the body.

Aim

To learn balance, the use of centre and grounding. To realign the legs, working the muscles of the feet and legs in a way that helps prevent rolling in and rolling out feet.

Preparation

▷ Stand sideways, close to a wall with your feet in parallel.

▷ Place a tennis ball between your ankles just below the inside ankle bone.

▷ Put one hand on the wall.

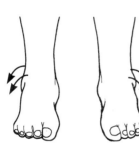

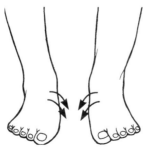

Avoid rolling the feet in and out

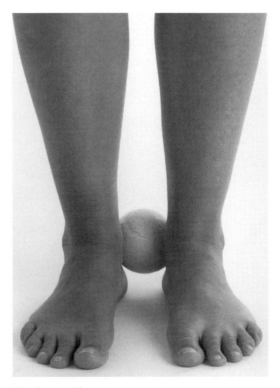

Starting position

Action

▷ Breathe in to prepare and lengthen up through the spine. Imagine that someone is pulling you up from the top of your head by a piece of string.

▷ Breathe out, navel to spine, and rise up on to the balls of your feet. Come right up, keeping the ball securely between the ankles. Your tailbone should be lengthening downwards so that your bottom does not stick out.

▷ Breathe in and lengthen upwards.

▷ Breathe out, navel to spine, and slowly come back down through the feet.

▷ Repeat eight times.

Awareness Points

▷ Keep lengthening up, up, up through the top of your head.

▷ Try to hold the wall in a way that does not make you twist your upper body.

▷ Do not stick your bottom out.

Variation

When you have mastered this you may add the following variation, checking all the time that your bottom is not sticking out.

When the feet are lowered back flat on the floor, bend your knees slightly, taking them directly over the feet (not between them or out to the sides), keep your heels on the floor, then slowly straighten them before you start the exercise again.

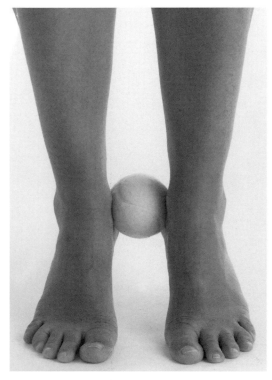

Rise up onto the balls of your feet

Balance

The human body can be likened to a very complicated machine. If **mechanical alignment** is good, the body will work very efficiently but no machine can work **efficiently** if it is not in balance, because **extra energy** must be spent to overcome the negative effects of any imbalance – its parts will start to wear out very quickly!

Balance

The most efficient use of the body is achieved if we have maximum output – that is, if movement is achieved from minimal muscular effort. We want just enough tension in a muscle to complete a task; no more, no less. For example, standing should not be tiring but it is for many people because their bodies are in poor postural alignment resulting in circulatory problems, undue stress on soft tissue and frequent and continued pressure of tight muscles on the veins of the lower limbs. With good alignment and use, only minimal muscular energy is required, there is minimal sagging against ligaments and only intermittent pressure on veins.

In the last chapters we introduced the three main body weights: the head, the ribcage and the pelvis. These weights are all interdependent, reacting to each other. When they are not stacked up in line on top of each other, muscles have to work very hard to keep the body upright.

The force of gravity acts at right angles to the earth and the body should be maintained perpendicular to the earth to support and balance it correctly with minimal strain and use of energy.

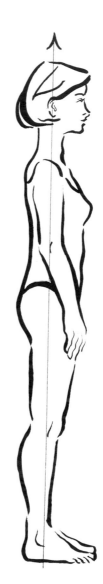

Starting with the feet as a base, the whole of the body should be aligned to achieve a natural balance. Ideally, none of these body weights should deviate too far from the vertical axis or plumbline. When the body is not balanced it is usually due to muscle weakness, which allows these weights to slip out of alignment. As a result, other muscles need to become very tight to keep the whole structure upright.

It is possible to say that muscle weakness and tightness can cause faulty alignment, causing the body to lose its natural balance. But we can also look at it from another viewpoint by saying that it is faulty alignment which causes muscles to be weak, tight or short. When muscles are chronically shortened the blood supply to this area is restricted, causing a variety of malfunctions. A balanced body, therefore, is one in which the weights are aligned correctly over each other and as close to the vertical plumbline as possible.

Throughout the book so far, we have been working towards correcting any muscle imbalances which you may have. In this chapter, we have included activities to help you achieve an overall sense of balance in your body.

Monkey

This is a smart way to use your body when you have to stand for any length of time, as it will relieve or prevent a stiff back. This is *not* a static position, for while in a 'Monkey' you have the maximum flexibility and mobility, it requires the minimum muscular effort.

In an ideal world we would use the 'Monkey' for almost all activities. While moving from sitting to standing (and vice versa) in a correct way we move through a 'Monkey'. Everyday activities such as bending, picking something up, lifting, standing at a work surface such as a kitchen sink should be performed with greater ease when using the 'Monkey'.

Preparation

▷ Stand with your feet slightly turned out, hip-width apart.

▷ Your weight should be evenly distributed on your feet.

▷ Let your neck be free of tension, so that your head can lengthen up. As a result your back will lengthen and also widen with every breath you take. Now you are ready.

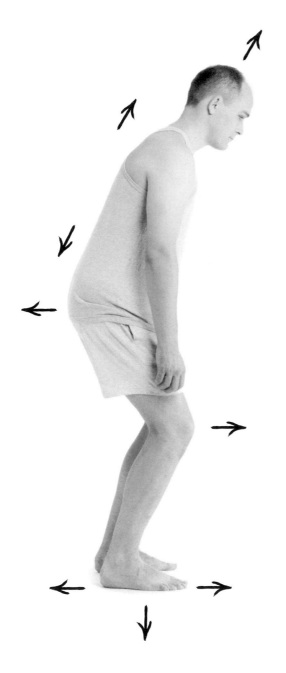

Action

▷ Tilt slightly forward from your hip joint, keeping your head, neck and back in one 'piece'.

▷ Pivot forward on the hip joint. At the same time, release your hips, knees and ankle joints to let the knees bend forwards. Make sure that your knees stay in alignment over your feet!

▷ Allow the back to widen and the arms to hang freely.

   Try not to think of bending down as this will probably trigger excessive muscular tension, especially in the hip flexors, thighs and ankles, which will restrict movement.

▷ Let your legs soften and bend – from that base your whole back is growing up.

▷ When coming back to an upright position, keep lengthening your back and head away and return to a balanced way of standing without 'locking' your knees.

Yin Yang Toner

The origins of this exercise lie not in the Pilates Method nor the Alexander Technique but rather within the Chinese medicine system. We have included it here because we have found that it really does boost the energy of our clients. We've even had our trainee teachers request to do this 'exercise' before their final theory examination – so it has the reputation of energizing the brain as well!

Chinese medicine has a fascinating way of seeing the body as a system of channels, invisible energy lines called meridians, through which the energy or Chi (pronounced 'chee') flows. This forms the basis for acupuncture, which has been in use for thousands of years as a treatment for rebalancing the body. You can compare the meridians to a system of pipes in a house When one of these pipes becomes blocked for whatever reason, the whole system is affected. Our body is very much the same, being a highly tuned and very complicated system in which all the parts react to each other and influence each other. Energy in our body needs to circulate and flow freely to maintain health and efficient use of the body.

The following Chi Kung exercise is based on the direction of the energy flow along the meridians and helps the energy to flow freely. Make sure that you follow the instructions carefully.

Aim

To energize and rebalance the body.

Action

▷ Stand comfortably, legs hip-width apart, toes facing forward, knees unlocked.

▷ Tap the top of your head with the tips of your fingers, keeping your hands, wrists and arms relaxed. The movement should be light and fluffy – imagine raindrops falling on your head.

▷ Repeat on the back of your neck.

▷ Stroke and rub your face, as if you were washing it.

▷ Pinch along the outside ridges of your ears.

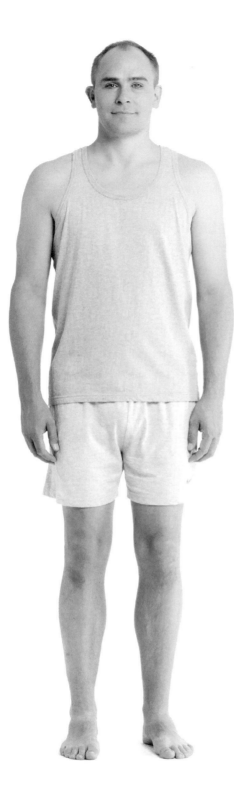

▷ Make a loose fist and tap down from your armpit to your hand along the inside of your arm. Continue back up on the outside, including the top of your shoulder.

▷ Repeat five times.

▷ Change arms. With the same loose fist, gently tap your breastbone about fifteen times.

▷ In a clockwise direction tap around your stomach. Start at the pubic bone and come up the right hand side and down the left side, following the direction of your digestive system.

▷ Repeat seven times.

▷ Gently bend your knees to tap down the outside of both legs and then back up on the inside. You can include your buttocks, the biggest muscle in the body.

▷ Repeat five times.

▷ Transfer your weight on to one leg, and tap the bottom of your foot.

▷ Repeat on the other side.

▷ Rub your hands together and then place them on your kidneys.

▷ Return to your starting position and be aware of any changes that have occurred during this exercise. Changes can include a feeling of warmth, tingling sensations, hot ears and an increased general energy level.

Balancing on One Leg

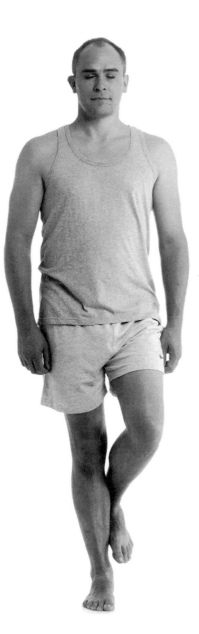

This exercise demonstrates clearly how much we rely on our visual sense to stay balanced. Without the visual messages to the brain, it has to rely on all the other senses.

We all tend to favour one leg which can grow stronger than its partner. This can have repercussions throughout the body. Exercises which require you to stand on one leg can help to strengthen the weaker leg. Don't worry if you do wobble around – the muscles of your ankles and feet get a great workout!

Aim

To learn to balance from within. To work the muscles of the ankles and feet. To work each leg individually.

Preparation

Stand in a balanced way, reminding yourself of all the directions given on page 50.

Action

▷ Breathe in and lengthen up through the spine.

▷ Breathe out, navel to spine, lift one leg off the floor and place it knee facing forward on the inside of the calf of your other leg.

▷ Find your balance.

▷ Now close your eyes.

▷ Breathe normally for five breaths.

▷ Repeat with the other leg.

Awareness Points

▷ Try not to sink into the hip of the leg you are standing on.

▷ Keep lengthening your waist.

Variation

There is a variation to this exercise using a tennis ball.

Following all the instructions given above to stand on one leg, try throwing and catching a tennis ball. You might like to do this in an empty room!

Keep your eyes open for this one!

Table Legs

Aim

To mobilize the spine, strengthen the abdominals and the gluteal muscles. To learn balance and control.

Preparation

Kneel on all fours, your hands directly beneath your shoulders, your knees beneath your hips. Check that your pelvis is neutral, the natural curve maintained.

Action

▷ Breathe in to prepare as you lengthen the spine from the top of your head to your tailbone.

▷ Breathe out, navel to spine, and slide the right leg away from you, straightening it along the floor.

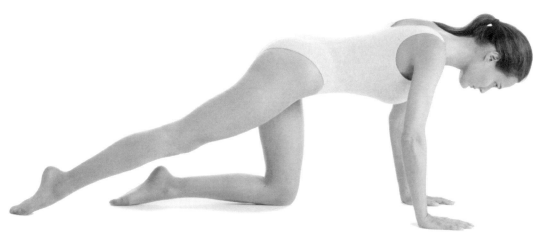

Leg straight but not lifted

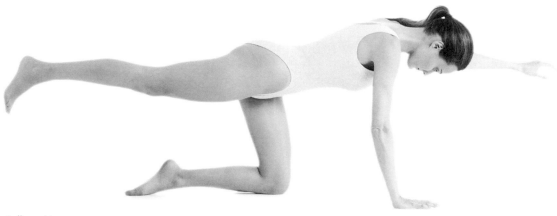

Full position

▷ When the leg is fully straight, lift it behind you to hip height – no higher! The pelvis stays square to the floor.

▷ Lift the *opposite*, left, arm and stretch it away from you at shoulder height. Look at the floor still, top of the head lengthening.

▷ Breathe in and lower the arm and leg.

▷ Repeat five times, alternating arms and legs.

Awareness Points

▷ Keep the lower abdominals engaged.

▷ Do not allow the pelvis to tilt to one side.

▷ Keep looking straight down at the floor – if you raise your head you will shorten the back of your neck.

When you can do this exercise easily, you can attempt the more advanced version on the next page.

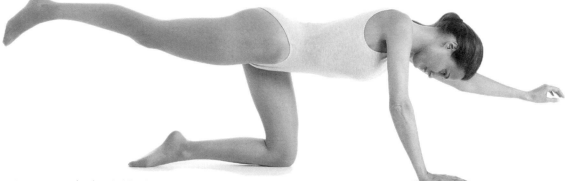

Incorrect – the leg is lifted too high and the pelvis is tilted

Advanced Table Legs

Preparation

Kneel on all fours, your hands directly beneath your shoulders, your knees beneath your hips. Check that your pelvis is neutral, the natural curve maintained.

Action

▷ Breathe in to prepare and lengthen from the top of your head to your tailbone.

▷ Breathe out, drawing the navel back to

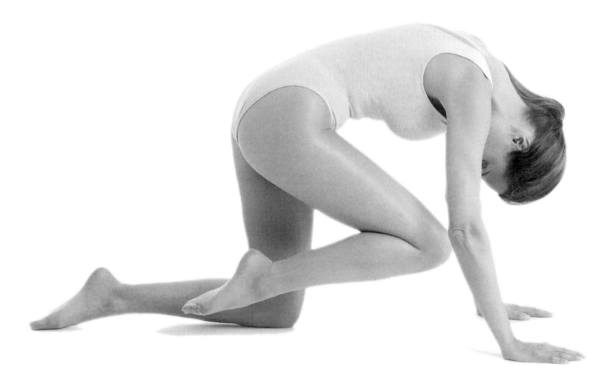

Head meeting knee

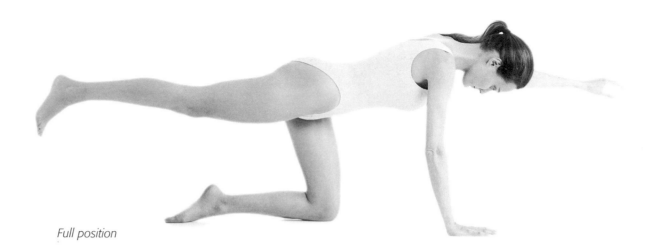

Full position

the spine and bring your right knee forward towards your head, curling your head to meet the knee while arching the back up.

▷ Breathe in while you are there.

▷ Breathe out, navel to spine, and straighten the leg behind you, extending it along the floor until the knee is straight, then lift the leg no higher than your buttocks. At the same time, lift your left arm and extend it in front of you. *Do not twist the pelvis – keep it square to you.*

▷ Breathe in and hold.

▷ Breathe out, navel to spine, and bend the knee in again, curling the head to meet it.

▷ Repeat five times on each side.

Directing:
Pathways

This is the last chapter in the book, bringing together all the **skills** that you have acquired. Through the explorations and exercises, the **neurological pathways** will have been used again and again, so that you should now be able to recognize them easily . . .

Directing: Pathways

Directing is somewhat like 'thinking' into the body, a thought alone being capable of bringing about tiny changes in the body. Sometimes those tiny changes can be enough to initiate the larger changes necessary towards a more balanced way of functioning. One of the discoveries made by Alexander was that the mere thought of a physical activity can 'trigger' certain physical changes in the body. He decided to base much of his new and innovative method on this fact. Pilates also recognized this and loved to quote Schiller: 'It is the mind itself which builds the body.' Pilates exercises are by their very nature 'thoughtful'.

'Thinking in' activity, 'thinking into' the body – inner body wisdom can be experienced as very strange at first. People quite often comment that they seem to be doing so little – or, even, nothing at all. It is those thoughts directed into the body, however, that will, over a period of time, sharpen the kinaesthetic sense It will then begin to function enough to provide reliable feedback.

The Pathways Cleared

In the past chapters, we have been exploring these neurological pathways that send messages from the brain via nerves to muscles, tendons and joints. Through the explorations and exercises, these pathways will have been used again and again, so that you should now be able to recognize them easily and have no problem accessing them swiftly when needed. Repeating simple movements with care and attention helps re-establish pathways and opens the way for more complex movements. Sending thoughts into your body or directing can be done anywhere, anytime and during any activity.

Once you have cleared those pathways and walked them time and again, the travelling becomes easier and a lot more fun!

Enjoy your body.

CASE STUDY

Sandra, a 30-year-old designer, came to Gordon Thompson of Body Control Pilates to reduce her upper body tension, tone her body and improve her general fitness. She was also concerned about the tension headaches she got from time to time.

Initially, she focused on strengthening core postural muscles and improved thoracic stabilization. She found weekly classes in the studio helped her to cope better with sitting at a desk all week – and this resulted in a noticeable reduction of her headaches. But after two years of gradual improvement, Sandra felt she had reached a plateau. She still had very distinct tension patterns, caused by an increased stress level at work. Gordon suggested Alexander Technique Lessons with Helge Fisher.

Initially, the Relaxation Position and focussing on her breathing slowed Sandra down and helped her on a daily basis. She found that taking the time to listen and explore the pathways inside her body gave her new insight into the way she usually reacted to stress. During even the first few weeks her tension was gradually released and she found it much easier to 'let go'.

Monkey on Toes

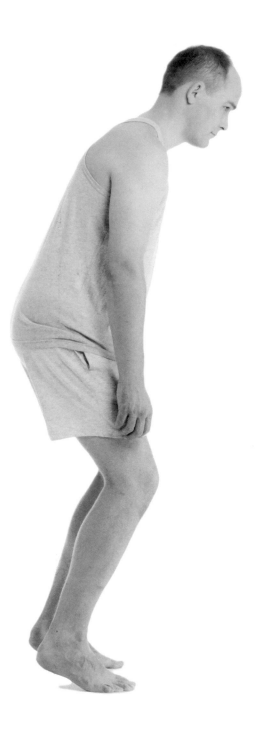

This exploration is an advanced version of the Monkey on page 148. It requires a balanced body and an ability to focus the mind.

    Please do not try this exercise until you have familiarized yourself with the Monkey position in everyday life.

Preparation

Adopt the Monkey position.

Action

▷ Bend your knees so that your body describes a zigzag in profile.

▷ Lengthen your back and lengthen your head away from your spine.

▷ Transfer your weight gradually over your toes and continue lengthening along the spine.

▷ Slowly, and in a controlled way, rise up on to your toes, still maintaining the Monkey position.

▷ On the way down, still keep the thought of lengthening away, while very slowly transferring your weight back on to the whole foot.

▷ Repeat this five times.

Awareness Points

▷ Make sure that you keep your knees and ankles in alignment, they are slightly turned out, hip-width apart.

▷ Move the whole back on the hip joint, like a hinge.

▷ Keep the back lengthened the whole time.

Chalk Circle Two

This exercise combines the movements of Side Rolls (page 124) with the original Chalk Circle (page 122). You should feel comfortable with both these before you attempt this version.

Before starting, you must read through the instructions several times as they are fairly complex. We suggest you add co-ordinating the breathing after you have perfected the movements.

Keep the navel firmly back to the spine throughout.

Please avoid this exercise if you have a disc-related injury

Aim

To open the upper body, stretching the tight pectoral muscles. To learn to initiate movements from a strong centre. To work the muscles of the waist and sides. To sense a 'release' of tension.

Preparation

Lie on your back with your knees bent, feet together and your head on a substantial pillow. Your arms are out to your sides.

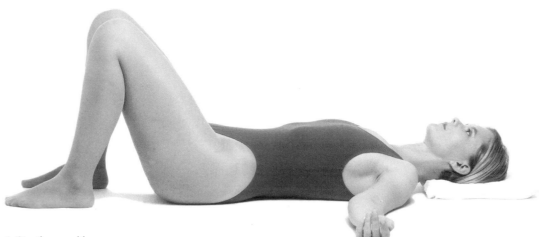

1. Starting position

Action

▷ Breathe in to prepare for movement.

▷ Breathe out, navel to spine, and roll your head and knees over to the left side, initiating the movement from your centre.

▷ At the same time, start to take your right arm down over your buttocks (photo 2) and across your body and up in a circular sweep past your left arm, towards your head, trying to keep contact with the floor.

▷ As your arm comes over your head, (photo 3) breathe in and, navel still back to spine, start to roll your knees back to centre and your head as well.

▷ As your arm descends down in a circle on your right side, breathe out and roll your knees to the right and your head as well.

▷ Now take your left arm down across your body, up past your right arm and over your head.

▷ Breathe in as the arm passes over above you on the floor, and breathe out as you bring the knees and head back to centre.

▷ Repeat five times to each side.

There are times when a video would come in handy! Please persevere for this exercise has one the best 'feel good' factors of any exercise we know.

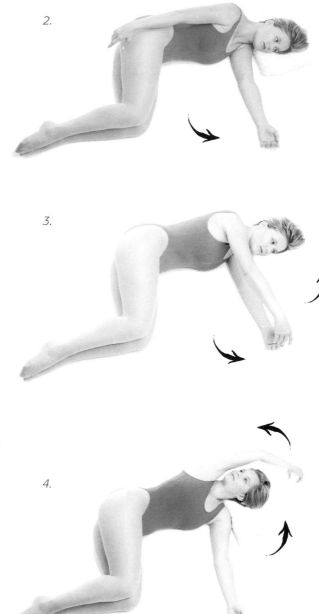

2.

3.

4.

Awareness Point

Keep your navel firmly back towards your spine throughout the exercise.

Pelvic Clocks

(renamed 'Beer Swills' by one thirsty client!)

We understand that this exercise has its origins in the Feldenkrais Method.

Aim

This exercise is a very gentle and useful way to familiarize yourself with the range of movement that is possible around your pelvic area and, so, be aware when it is out of alignment. It especially highlights where the muscles are tight and, therefore, restricting movement.

Preparation

Adopt the Relaxation Position.

Action

▷ First, make sure that you are in a neutral pelvis position.

▷ Imagine a clock face on your stomach. Your pubic bone is 6 o'clock, your navel 12 o'clock. Visualize a marble on that clockface. By gently tilting your pelvis, let that marble roll from 12 o'clock to 1 o'clock, to 2 o'clock right around the clock until you reach 12 o'clock again.

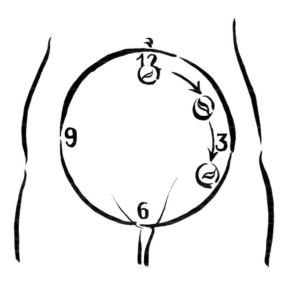

You will possibly notice that your movements are very easy and smooth in some areas, other areas are tight and it seems quite an effort to make the marble go round the perimeters. Commonly, we find that around 7 o'clock to 9 o'clock are tighter than the rest.

▷ Try this clockwise and, then, also anti-clockwise!

Once you are more familiar with 'pelvic clocks' in the Relaxation Position, you can also try them:

▷ Lying on your side in a foetal position (as in the Chalk Circle, page 122).

▷ On all fours

▷ Standing with bent knees, feet hip-width apart

▷ Sitting in a chair

Awareness Points

▷ Try to keep the movements small and controlled.

▷ Avoid gripping in the thighs or moving the legs around.

Diamond Press

(includes the Rest Position)

Although not a dramatic exercise to watch, if you can feel that connection between the shoulderblades and the small of your back, you can also feel the neck grow a couple of inches as it is freed. This is great for reversing the effects of being 'hunched over' all day.

Aim

To work the mid-back muscles, allowing the neck to release. To develop awareness of the scapulae. To encourage lengthening while extending the back.

Preparation

▷ Lie on your front with your feet hip-width apart and parallel.

▷ Create a diamond shape with your arms by placing your fingertips together just above your forehead. Your elbows are open, your shoulder blades relaxed.

Action

▷ Breathe in and lengthen through the spine.

▷ Breathe out, navel to spine, and pull the shoulderblades down into the back of your waist. Your head lifts an inch or two off the floor, but you stay looking at the floor, the back of the neck long. Imagine a cord pulling you from the top of your head. Really make the connection down into the small of your back – you have to push a little on the elbows, but think of

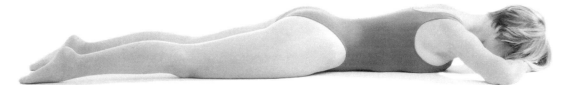

Starting position

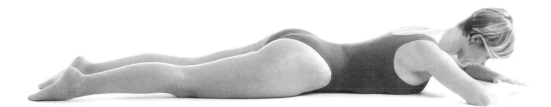

Full position – side view

them connecting with your waist as well.

Keep the lower stomach lifted but the ribs on the floor.

▷ Breathe in and slowly lower.

▷ Repeat five times.

Awareness Points

▷ Keep the navel to spine.

▷ Look down at the floor – if you lift your head you will shorten the back of the neck.

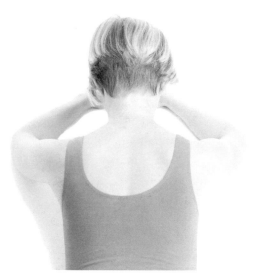

Full position – from above

The Rest Postition

When you have completed the repetitions, come back to sit on your heels. Your knees are apart, your feet together. Stretch out the muscles you have just been working. If you have a knee injury simply curl up on your side.

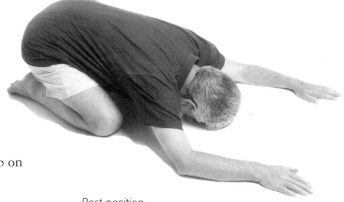

Rest position

Single Leg Stretch

This is a superb exercise, which combines all the 8 Principles of Pilates in a complex movement sequence. It is an advanced exercise, so only attempt it when you are stronger.

Please lower the head if the neck feels strained in this exercise. If you have a neck problem or if you find that you are straining the neck, use a pillow or wedge to support the head and neck.

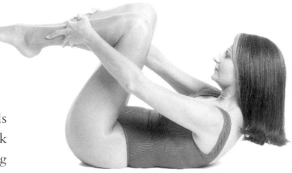

Starting position

Aim

To improve co-ordination in the body. To sense lengthening out from the centre. To strengthen the abdominal muscles. To work the hip flexors. To work the deep neck flexors.

Preparation

▷ Lie on the mat, draw your knees up on to your chest, the toes just touching – but not the heels. Keep your feet softly pointed.

▷ Place your hands on the outside of your calves.

▷ Your elbows are open to enable the chest to expand fully.

Action

▷ Breathe in as you soften the breastbone, and slowly curl your head, neck and shoulders off the floor to look at your stomach – keep a gap under your chin, though. Leave your head on the pillow, if using one.

▷ Breathe out and, anchoring navel to spine, move the left hand to hold the inside of the right knee and stretch your left leg away in parallel, so that it

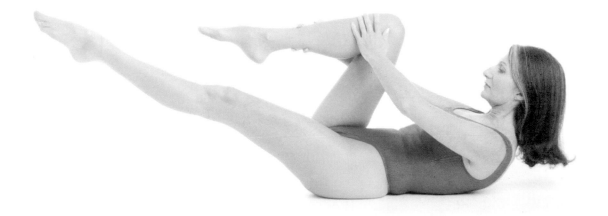

is at an angle of 45 degrees to the floor. The toes are softly pointed.

▷ Breathe in wide, as you begin to bend the leg back on to your chest, bringing it back into your shoulder.

▷ Change the hands so that, now, your left hand is on the outside of your left leg, your right hand on the inside of your left knee.

▷ Breathe out, checking the navel is still pulled back to the spine as you now extend the right leg.

▷ Breathe in wide as the leg bends back into your shoulder.

▷ Repeat ten times with each leg.

Awareness Points

▷ Try to keep the torso square, or, more appropriately, rectangular – don't let one side collapse downwards.

▷ When you first attempt this exercise,

make sure that one knee is safely bent and held before the other is extended. As you become more familiar with the movements, you can make the hand exchange and leg stretch simultaneous.

▷ At no time should there be any daylight under your back. Keep it firmly anchored to the floor. If you find that your back is arching, then raise the angle of the extended leg.

▷ Check that your shoulderblades are down into your back.

▷ Allow the chin to be gently rotated towards your chest, but not tucked in, so that the neck remains long.

▷ If you cannot reach your ankle, then hold the side of your shin.

▷ Once you have extended the leg, keep the angle constant.

This exercise can also be done turning the extended leg out from the hip joint.

The Advanced Version: Oblique Leg Stretch

Aim

To work the oblique muscles.

Preparation

▷ Lie on your back, draw your knees up on to your chest, the toes just touching – but not the heels.

▷ Keep your feet softly pointed.

▷ Clasp your hands behind your head. The elbows stay open.

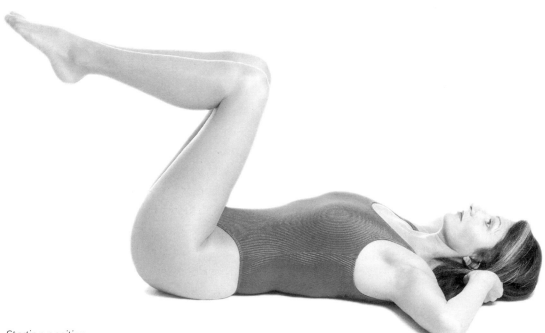

Starting position

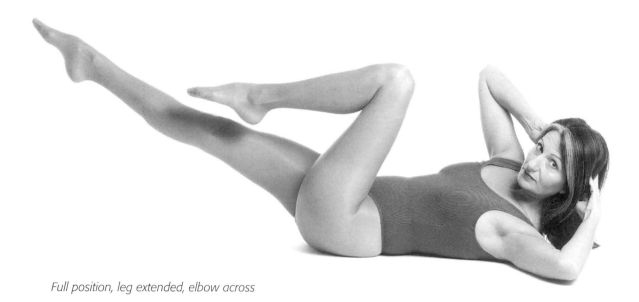

Full position, leg extended, elbow across

Action

▷ Breathe in to prepare.

▷ Breathe out, navel to spine as you curl up, softening the breastbone and taking the right shoulder in the direction of your left knee. The upper body stays open, the elbows in line. The right leg straightens as it extends away in parallel.

▷ Breathe in as the knee bends back and you return to the floor.

▷ Breathe out, navel to spine and curl the left shoulder towards the right bent knee, extending the left leg away.

▷ Breathe in as the knee bends back and the left shoulder returns to the floor.

▷ Repeat ten times to each side.

This exercise can also be done without lowering the upper body back to the floor each time. Stay curled up off the floor and rotate the upper body, alternately bringing opposite shoulder to the bent knee.

Awareness Points

Make sure that the shoulder, and not the elbow, comes across towards the bent knee. Keep the elbows in line, do not allow them to come forward – it is your shoulder that is directed towards the knee. In this way, the upper body stays open.

Scissors Preparation

Aim

To be able to move the limbs while maintaining a strong centre (core stability), the back secure and the neck released.

Preparation

▷ Lie on the mat, and bring your knees on to your chest one at a time.
▷ Take hold of the left leg with both hands, behind the thigh and hold it securely to you, keeping the elbows open, the neck soft, the shoulderblades down into your back.

Action

▷ Breathe in to prepare.
▷ Breathe out, hollowing navel to spine, and straighten the right leg up into the air.

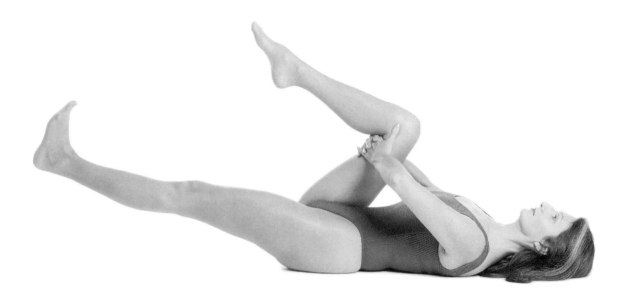

▷ Breathe in and flex the right foot down towards your face, lengthening through the heel.

▷ Breathe out, navel to spine, and lower the leg to the floor, lengthening the whole time through the heel . . . a long, long leg.

▷ Breathe in as the foot rests on the floor.

▷ Breathe out, navel to spine, and raise the straight leg up again.

▷ Change arms and legs.

▷ Repeat five times with each leg.

Awareness Points

▷ Navel to spine throughout, tailbone down and lengthening away.

▷ Check constantly that your upper body is soft and open, the elbows open, the breastbone soft.

▷ Your shoulder blades stay down into your back.

▷ The legs are to be as straight as possible.

The Full Scissors

When you can do the last exercise and the Single Leg Stretch easily, you may attempt the Full Scissors. It is an advanced exercise, so please stop if it feels uncomfortable. You need stretched hamstrings to do this properly, so be sure to warm up with the Beach Ball Hamstrings (page 94) first.

Preparation

▷ Lie on the mat. Your knees are both bent on to your chest.
▷ Take hold of the right leg behind the thigh.

Action

▷ Breathe in to prepare.
▷ Breathe out, navel to spine, and raise your head and shoulders off the floor. Keep a soft breastbone.

▷ Breathe in and straighten both legs up into the air, the toes softly pointed – you still have hold of the right leg behind the thigh.
▷ Breathe out, navel firmly to spine, and lengthen the left leg down towards the floor, stopping just above it.
▷ Breathe in and raise the left leg as straight as possible.
▷ Breathe out and change arms and legs, lowering the right leg now.
▷ Aim to make the legs cross over like scissors. Your back should stay firmly anchored throughout, navel to spine. The legs are as straight as possible. You should be breathing out as the leg lowers down, in, as it starts to raise, out, as the other leg lowers.

▷ Scissor the legs twenty times. Then slowly lower the head down.

Awareness Points

Breathing deeply into your lower ribcage, check constantly that:

your upper body is soft and open
the elbows are open
the breastbone is soft
your shoulderblades are down into your back
you maintain navel to spine throughout
the legs are as straight as possible
the legs are kept parallel and in a line with your hips

The Glass Table

Aim

To learn to stabilize the spine while performing large movements with the legs. To increase awareness for the sides of your body. To learn to move the leg at the same level, in the same plane, through space, maintaining stability in the pelvis.

Preparation

▷ Lie on your right side, with your right arm stretched out in a line with your body.

▷ Let your head rest on your right arm and look straight ahead – use a small flat cushion under your ear if more comfortable.

▷ Check that your body is in a straight line. You might like to use a wall to lie against as a reference point – not to lean into, though.

▷ Then, bend both your legs at the hip joint, keeping the knees straight, until they are at a 40 degree angle to the torso.

▷ Place your left hand on the floor opposite your chest to steady your torso, making sure that you keep your shoulders relaxed and down.

▷ Make sure that both hip bones are directly on top of each other and check that you are not twisting in the pelvis.

An advanced version

When you can accomplish the above easily, after bringing the leg forward, you may try taking the top leg back in line with your body – not behind it – before returning it to rest on the underneath leg.

Action

▷ Breathe in to prepare, release the neck and lengthen up through the spine.

▷ Breathe out, navel to spine, and lift the top leg to hip level – about 15 centimetres (6 inches) off the floor.

▷ Breathe in, checking that your waist has not sunk into the floor.

▷ Breathe out, navel to spine, and bring the leg forward without changing the alignment in your back, especially the lower back. A good image is that you are sliding your leg across a glass table. Keep the abdominals strong and only bring the leg as far forward as you can without losing the position of your back.

▷ Breathe in and then breathe out, navel still firmly back to spine, bring the leg back above your underneath leg and lower it to rest.

▷ Repeat five times on both sides.

Awareness Points

▷ Keep lifting your waist off the floor and keep lengthening in your body, so that you do not sink into the floor.

▷ Keep the image of the glass table so that the leg does not drop.

▷ Be completely aware of your lower back and pelvis throughout. It must stay stable, supported by strong abdominals.

Sessions

Rather than simply dividing the exercises into daily workouts, we thought it might be fun to group them together so that they not only provide a balanced session, but they are mood enhancing as well!

In order to get a well-rounded fitness programme, you should aim to practice three times a week and include all the sessions below in a one-month period.

De-stresser

Had a bad day? Try the following exercises and feel your tensions evaporate. Concentrating on the pathways from your mind to your body is one of the best ways to unwind.

Relaxation Position (page 46)

Tense and Release (page 52)

Navel to Spine Arms/Legs/Opposite (page 35)

Pelvic Floor, Elevator and Flower (pages 77, 78, 79)

Spine Curl with Breath (page 108)

Side Rolls (page 124)

Chalk Circle (page 122)

Beach Ball Hamstrings (page 94)

Diamond Press (page 168)

Quadriceps Lengthening (page 85)

Rest Position (page 169)

Single Leg Stretch (page 170)

Floating Shoulders (page 70)

Foot Massage (page 132)

Standing Like a Tree (page 134)

Roll Downs (page 58)

Melting Body (page 92)

Energizing and Invigorating

Perhaps you feel a little sluggish in the mornings and just can't seem to get going. These exercises will improve your flow of energy and circulation. The perfect start to the day!

Yin Yang Toner (page 150)

Pelvic Clocks (page 166)

Curl Ups (page 98)

Oblique Curl Ups (page 100)

Wall Curls (page 86)

Ankle Circles (page 138)

Twister (page 104)

The Big Squeeze (page 80)

Table Legs (or Advanced Table Legs) (pages 154, 156)

Beach Ball Hamstrings (page 94)

Adductor Openings (page 84)

Scissors (Preparation or Full) (pages 174, 176)

The Glass Table (page 178)

Chalk Circle (page 122)

Opening Doors (page 72)
Monkey (page 148)
Roll Downs (page 58)

Balancing

We all feel unbalanced at times, not just physically, but mentally and emotionally as well. Sometimes things seem to be growing out of proportion. That important decision you are supposed to make by Friday is hanging over you and you are no nearer to reaching it. Or perhaps you found yourself flying off the handle this morning because you couldn't find the other matching sock! Try this workout and clear the mind, restore the balance.

Standing Like a Tree (page 134)
Yin Yang Toner (page 150)
Relaxation Position (page 46)
Pelvic Clocks (page 166)
Knee Bends (page 62)
Zigzags (page 60)
Curl Ups with a Scarf (page 102)
Single Leg Stretch (page 170)
Diamond Press (page 168)
Quadriceps Lengthening (page 85)
Rest Position (page 169)
The Emergency Stop (page 79)
Sunbathing Spider (page 56)
Triceps Stretch (page 96)
Grounding while Sitting (page 136)
Balancing on One Leg (page 152)
Monkey (page 148)

Calming

Can't sleep? Maybe your mind is still racing and your adrenaline pumping. The follow-ing have a very calming effect on the ner-vous system and so are an ideal way to switch off at the end of the day.

Relaxation Position (page 46)
Tense and Release (page 52)
Use of Centre – Co-ordinating Arms and Legs (page 120)
Spine Curl with Breath (page 108)
Cherry Picking (page 140)
Chalk Circle (page 122)
Grounding while Sitting (page 136)
Beach Ball Hamstrings (page 94)
Pelvic Roll Backs (page 126)
Figure of Eight (page 77)
Table Legs (page 154)
Single or Oblique Leg Stretch (page 170 or 172)
Roll Downs (page 58)
The Pillow Squeeze (page 82)
Tennis Ball Massage (page 137)
Sunbathing Spider (page 56)

Rejuvenating

Some days you quite simply feel your age – and more! How on earth are you going to summon up the energy to go to that party after work *and* look good into the bargain? Exercise the life back into your body with this wonderful pick-me-up routine.

Yin Yang Toner (page 150)
Relaxation Position (page 46)
Zigzags (page 60)
Wall Curls (page 86)
Curl Ups with a Scarf (page 102)
Beach Ball Hamstrings (page 94)
Side Rolls (page 124)
Single Leg Stretch (page 170)
Scissors (Preparation or Full) (pages 174, 176)

Shoulder Presses (page 74)

Pelvic Elevator (page 78)

Tennis Ball Massage (page 137)

Big Squeeze (page 80)

Diamond Press (page 168)

Quadriceps Lengthening (page 85)

Rest Position (page 169)

Advanced Table Legs (page 156)

Roll Downs (page 58)

We have also given you sessions to do before and after sport or a gym workout. Obviously, you will need a mat to practice on – a muddy football pitch or gravel tennis court will not do!

Before Sport

It isn't just the muscles that need warming up and preparing before sport – it's the mind as well. This short warm-up programme has been designed not only to help you avoid injury, but also to provide enormous psychological benefits. If your sport is a competitive one, these mind body exercises will help you focus into the bargain.

Use of Centre – Co-ordinating Arms and Legs (page 120)

Beach Ball Hamstrings (page 94)

Spine Curls – Hip Flexor Stretch (page 110)

Side Rolls (page 124)

Curl Ups with a Scarf (page 102)

Adductor Openings (page 84)

Ankle Circles (page 138)

Diamond Press (page 168)

Quadriceps Lengthening (page 85)

Rest Position (page 169)

Triceps Stretch (page 96)

Roll Downs (page 58)

After Sport

A lot of sports require you to use certain muscles repeatedly while totally ignoring others. You only have to think of the way you play tennis to see how easily the body can become one-sided and unbalanced. This after-sport session will help to correct any such body imbalances and will also help to prevent you feeling sore the next day. Skip it at your peril!

Navel to Spine – Full Stretch (page 33)

Pelvic Clocks (page 166)

Beach Ball Hamstrings (page 94)

Pelvic Roll Backs (page 126)

Cherry Picking (page 140)

Table Legs – Rest Position (page 171)

Roll Downs (page 58)

Chalk Circle (either) (page 122 or 164)

The Pillow Squeeze (page 82)

Relaxation Position (page 46)

The next two sessions include exercises which are particularly helpful if you are pregnant or if you have a back problem. Please check with your medical practitioner before you attempt them.

Pregnancy

The benefits of continuing to do some form of exercise during pregnancy are now well accepted. Mothers need to be fit not just for the birth, but also for the strenuous times to follow! Furthermore, a lot of expectant mums suffer from chronic backache during pregnancy which can be prevented with the right type of exercise. But what *is* the right type of exercise? Pilates fits the bill perfectly, as it gently brings the body into correct alignment and safely strengthens the muscles needed to maintain good posture and to facilitate an easier birth.

The body undergoes a great many changes during pregnancy and, for obvious reasons, great care must be taken when exercising. We strongly advise against doing these exercises during the first 6 to 14 weeks of your pregnancy, and you should take care not to lie on your back for longer than five minutes after your second trimester.

You should consult a qualified medical practitioner before embarking on this programme. Listen closely to your own body as you exercise – you should feel no discomfort at all, however, you will probably find the Relaxation Position uncomfortable from the second trimester.

Pelvic Floor exercises(page 76) – please note the advice on page 72.

Chalk Circle 1, (page 122)

Adductor Openings (page 84)

Ankle Circles (page 138)

Cherry Picking (page 140)

Triceps Stretch (page 96)

Shoulder Presses (page 74)

Opening Doors (page 72)

Twister – on a chair (page 104)

Grounding while Sitting (page 136)

While doing the next two exercises please pay special attention to keeping your pelvis square:

Table Legs (page 154)

The Glass Table (a cushion under your bump, if necessary) (page 178)

Tennis Ball Massage (page 137)

Monkey (page 148)

Back Problems

There are many different causes of back problems, and it is sensible to take medical advice before you begin to exercise. However, the days when you were told to stay in bed and take painkillers should be long gone! There's a lot you can do to help yourself and we have found the following session to be a favourite among back-pain sufferers. As always, approach the exercises with due care and attention and build up your strength and flexibility gradually.

Relaxation Position (page 46)

Use of Centre – all of these exercises as well as those on page 33 in 'Some Basic Rules to Good Body Use'

Pillow Squeeze (page 82)

Big Squeeze (page 80)

The Pelvic Floor (page 76)

Adductor Openings (page 84)

Spine Curls with Breath (page 108)

Hip Flexor (page 110)

Diamond Press (not too high) (page 168)

Quadriceps Lengthening (page 85)

Rest Position (page 169)

Table Legs (page 154)

Opening Doors (page 72)

Triceps Stretch (page 96)

Shoulder Presses (page 74)

Side Rolls – not if there are disc-related problems (page 124)

Tennis Ball Massage (page 137)

Grounding while Sitting (page 136)

Melting Body (page 92)

Bibliography

The following publications have been invaluable to the authors both as a source of information and inspiration in the writing of this book:

Your Body, Biofeedback at its Best
B.J. Jencks, Nelson Hall, Chicago, 1977

'Muscle Control – Pain Control. What exercises would you prescribe?'
Article by C.A. Richardson and G.A. Jull, Department of Physiotherapy, University of Queensland, Australia. *Manual Therapy*, Pearson Professional Ltd., 1995

'Dysfunction of Tranversus Abdominus associated with Chronic Low Back Pain. Article by P.W. Hodges, Department of Physiotherapy, University of Queensland, Australia. *MPAA Conference Proceedings*, 1995

Manual of Structural Kinesiology
Clem Thompson, Times Mirror / Mosby College Publishing, 1989

Anatomy of Movement
Blandine Calais-Germain, Eastland Press, 1993

The Anatomy Coloring Book
Wynn Kapit and Lawrence M. Elson, HarperCollins Publishers, 1977

Inside Ballet Technique
Valerie Grieg, Princeton Book Company, 1994

Dancing Longer, Dancing Stronger
Andrea Watkins and Priscilla M. Clarkson, Princeton Book Company, 1990

Flexibility, Principles and Practice
Christopher Norris, Black, 1994

Dance Kinesiology
Sally Sevey Fitt, Schirmer, 1988

The Body Has Its Reasons: Anti-Exercises and Self-Awareness
Therese Bertherat and Carol Bernstein, Cedar, 1988

The Art Of Changing – A New Approach to the Alexander Technique
Glen Park, Ashgrove Press Ltd., 1989

Back Trouble – A New Approach to Prevention and Recovery
Deborah Caplan, Triad Publishing, 1987

Therapeutic Exercise Foundations and Techniques
Carolyn Kisner and Lynn Allen Colby, F.A. Davis Company, 1990

Human Movement Potential – Its Ideokinetic Facilitation
Lulu Swiegard, Harper and Row Publishers Inc., University Press of America Inc., 1974

Body Stories – A Guide To Experiential Anatomy
Andrea Olsen, Station Hill Press, 1991

Body Fitness and Exercise – Basic Theory and Practice for Therapists
Mo Rosser, Hodder and Stoughton, 1995

Sports Injuries – Diagnosis and Management for Physiotherapists
Christopher Norris, Butterworth Heinemann, 1993

Muscle Testing and Function
Kendall, Kendall and Wadsworth, Williams and Wilkins, Baltimore/London, 1971

Creative Visualisation
Shakti Gawain, Bantam Books, 1979

On Pilates:

Body Control : The Pilates Way
Lynne Robinson and Gordon Thomson, Boxtree, London, 1997

How to Improve Your Posture
Fran Lehen, Cornerstone Library, 1982

The Pilates Method of Physical and Mental Conditioning
Philip Friedman and Gail Eisen, Warner Books, 1980

Every Body is Beautiful
Ron Fletcher, Lippencott, 1974

For Further Information

 For a list of Pilates teachers and teacher training programmes send a stamped addressed envelope to:

The Body Control Pilates Association
17 Queensberry Mews West
South Kensington
London, SW7 2DY

 For information on books, videos, workshops, equipment and clothing, send an s.a.e. to:

Body Control Pilates Ltd
P.O. Box 238
Tonbridge
Kent TN11 8ZL

 Regular information updates appear on the Body Control Pilates website at **www.bodycontrol.co.uk**

Other useful addresses

**The Society of Teachers of the
Alexander Technique
(Worldwide Membership)
10 London House, 266 Fulham Road,
London, SW10 9EL**

The Physicalmind Institute
1807 Second Street # 28, Santa Fe,
New Mexico 87501, USA

The Australian Pilates Method Association
PO Box 27, Mosman, NSW 2088, Australia

*The following organizations may also
be useful:*

Osteopathic Information Service
PO Box 2074, Reading, Berkshire,
RG1 4YR

The Chartered Society of Physiotherapy
14 Bedford Row, London, WC1R 4ED

The Exercise Association of England Ltd.
Unit 4, Angel Gate, 326 City Road, London
EC1V 2PT

The National Back Pain Association
16 Elmtree Rd, Teddington, Middlesex
TW11 8ST

Holistic Massage Courses
The Academy of Natural Health
7a Clapham Common Southside,
London SW4 7AA

BODY CONTROL: The Pilates Way

Lynne Robinson & Gordon Thomson

'For more than 60 years, Pilates has been the best kept secret of the fit, the chic and the beautiful.' *The Times*

Pilates, 'the exercise world's best-kept secret', has won widespread acclaim and popularity through the success of Lynne Robinson and Gordon Thomson's first book, *Body Control*.

This number one health and exercise best-seller is the classic Pilates manual for the layperson. It introduces this unique system through 40 exercises, with programmed combinations, and is fully illustrated with photographs and muscle or joint explanations.

As featured on GMTV, *This Morning* and BBC2's *Looking Good*.

Pan Books are proud to continue publishing Body Control Pilates into the new millennium. Ask your local bookshop for details of the latest book from these authors!

Body Control: The Pilates Way
Demy pb   0330 369458   £7.99

Now available as a Pan book from your local bookshop or by sending a cheque or postal order payable to:

Book Services By Post
PO Box 29
Douglas
Isle of Man
IM99 1BQ

Or call 01624 675137 with a major credit card number.

Postage and packing free.

Praise for **BODY CONTROL:** The Pilates Way

'Pilates gave me a better understanding of the way exercise is not about how you look to others but how you feel about yourself. Pilates shows that the way to achieve this is to train the mind to control the body.' **Cheryl Homes Perfect,** *Sunday Times*

'There was no area of my life that didn't improve radically.' **Simon Callow**

'An excellent book to recommend.' *Physiotherapy*

'Pilates is a fundamental part of my dance training.' **Wayne Sleep**

'I used muscles in Pilates I never knew I had . . .' *Cosmopolitan*

'I believe the sports world has much to learn from Pilates exercises.' **Sharron Davies**

'Pilates is anatomically based; you have to be aware of what each muscle is doing . . . it shares mind and body control.' *Daily Telegraph*

'There are three things I trust: The Lord, my family and body control!' **Patti Boulaye**

'Astonishing results – this method delivers its promises.' **Consultant Osteopath Piers Chandler, DO, MRO**

'The perfect way to introduce a beginner to the Pilates method.' **Pat Cash**

'As a dancer, Pilates helps to strengthen and tone; as a singer, Pilates helps to correct posture and breathing; and if I am ever injured and unable to train fully, Pilates helps to maintain fitness while I am recuperating and repairing.' **Bonnie Langford**

'A relaxing, strengthening, graceful relief.' **Tracy Ulman**

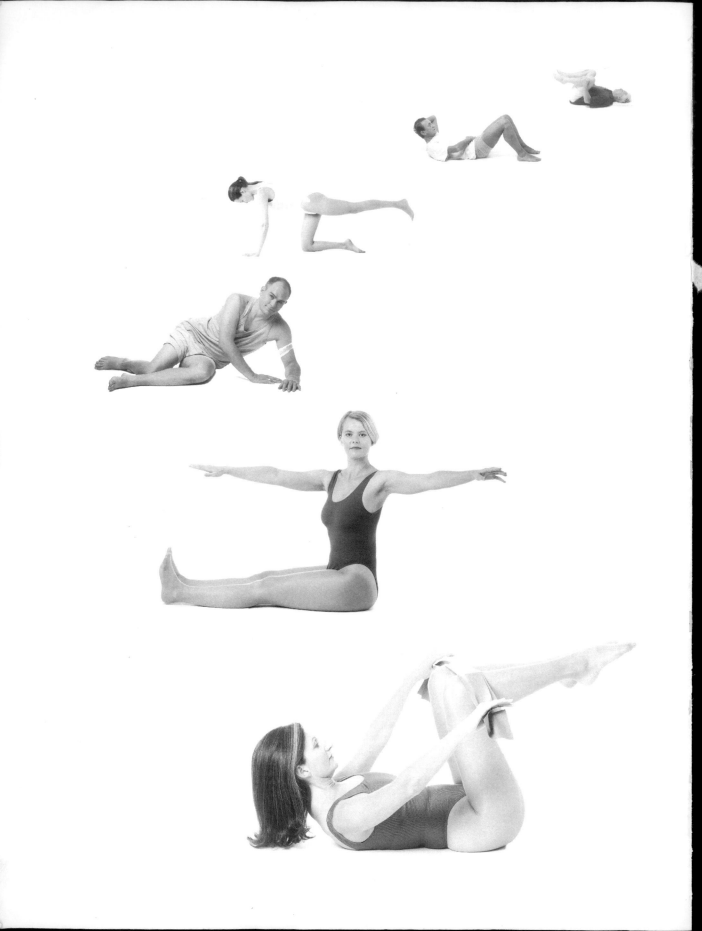